Prevention | 2026
CALENDAR AND HEALTH PLANNER

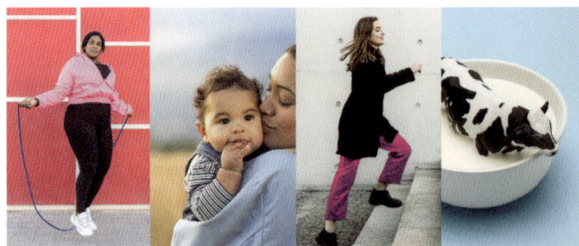

Phases of the Moon

● New moon ◑ First quarter ○ Full moon ◐ Last quarter

This planner is intended as a reference volume only, not as a medical manual. The information given here is designed to help you make informed decisions about your health. It is not intended as a substitute for any treatment that may have been prescribed by your doctor. If you suspect that you have a medical problem, we urge you to seek competent medical help.

The information in this planner is meant to supplement, not replace, proper exercise training. All forms of exercise pose some inherent risks. The editors and publisher advise readers to take full responsibility for their safety and know their limits. Before practicing the exercises in this planner, be sure that your equipment is well maintained, and do not take risks beyond your level of experience, aptitude, training, and fitness. The exercise and dietary programs in this planner are not intended as a substitute for any exercise routine or dietary regimen that may have been prescribed by your doctor. As with all exercise and dietary programs, you should get your doctor's approval before beginning.

Mention of specific companies, organizations, or authorities in this planner does not imply endorsement by the author or publisher, nor does mention of specific companies, organizations, or authorities imply that they endorse this planner, its author, or the publisher. Internet addresses and telephone numbers given in this planner were accurate at the time it went to press.

Printed in China

Planner design by Carol Angstadt
Photo editing by Monica Matthews
Photo credits can be found on the last page of the planner.

ISBN-13: 978-1-955710-42-8   hardcover
2 4 6 8 10 9 7 5 3 1   hardcover

HEARST

2025

SEPTEMBER
M	T	W	T	F	S	S
1	2	3	4	5	6	7
8	9	10	11	12	13	14
15	16	17	18	19	20	21
22	23	24	25	26	27	28
29	30					

OCTOBER
M	T	W	T	F	S	S
		1	2	3	4	5
6	7	8	9	10	11	12
13	14	15	16	17	18	19
20	21	22	23	24	25	26
27	28	29	30	31		

NOVEMBER
M	T	W	T	F	S	S
					1	2
3	4	5	6	7	8	9
10	11	12	13	14	15	16
17	18	19	20	21	22	23
24	25	26	27	28	29	30

DECEMBER
M	T	W	T	F	S	S
1	2	3	4	5	6	7
8	9	10	11	12	13	14
15	16	17	18	19	20	21
22	23	24	25	26	27	28
29	30	31				

2026

JANUARY
M	T	W	T	F	S	S
			1	2	3	4
5	6	7	8	9	10	11
12	13	14	15	16	17	18
19	20	21	22	23	24	25
26	27	28	29	30	31	

FEBRUARY
M	T	W	T	F	S	S
						1
2	3	4	5	6	7	8
9	10	11	12	13	14	15
16	17	18	19	20	21	22
23	24	25	26	27	28	

MARCH
M	T	W	T	F	S	S
						1
2	3	4	5	6	7	8
9	10	11	12	13	14	15
16	17	18	19	20	21	22
23	24	25	26	27	28	29
30	31					

APRIL
M	T	W	T	F	S	S
		1	2	3	4	5
6	7	8	9	10	11	12
13	14	15	16	17	18	19
20	21	22	23	24	25	26
27	28	29	30			

MAY
M	T	W	T	F	S	S
				1	2	3
4	5	6	7	8	9	10
11	12	13	14	15	16	17
18	19	20	21	22	23	24
25	26	27	28	29	30	31

JUNE
M	T	W	T	F	S	S
1	2	3	4	5	6	7
8	9	10	11	12	13	14
15	16	17	18	19	20	21
22	23	24	25	26	27	28
29	30					

JULY
M	T	W	T	F	S	S
		1	2	3	4	5
6	7	8	9	10	11	12
13	14	15	16	17	18	19
20	21	22	23	24	25	26
27	28	29	30	31		

AUGUST
M	T	W	T	F	S	S
					1	2
3	4	5	6	7	8	9
10	11	12	13	14	15	16
17	18	19	20	21	22	23
24	25	26	27	28	29	30
31						

SEPTEMBER
M	T	W	T	F	S	S
	1	2	3	4	5	6
7	8	9	10	11	12	13
14	15	16	17	18	19	20
21	22	23	24	25	26	27
28	29	30				

OCTOBER
M	T	W	T	F	S	S
			1	2	3	4
5	6	7	8	9	10	11
12	13	14	15	16	17	18
19	20	21	22	23	24	25
26	27	28	29	30	31	

NOVEMBER
M	T	W	T	F	S	S
						1
2	3	4	5	6	7	8
9	10	11	12	13	14	15
16	17	18	19	20	21	22
23	24	25	26	27	28	29
30						

DECEMBER
M	T	W	T	F	S	S
	1	2	3	4	5	6
7	8	9	10	11	12	13
14	15	16	17	18	19	20
21	22	23	24	25	26	27
28	29	30	31			

2027

JANUARY
M	T	W	T	F	S	S
				1	2	3
4	5	6	7	8	9	10
11	12	13	14	15	16	17
18	19	20	21	22	23	24
25	26	27	28	29	30	31

FEBRUARY
M	T	W	T	F	S	S
1	2	3	4	5	6	7
8	9	10	11	12	13	14
15	16	17	18	19	20	21
22	23	24	25	26	27	28

MARCH
M	T	W	T	F	S	S
1	2	3	4	5	6	7
8	9	10	11	12	13	14
15	16	17	18	19	20	21
22	23	24	25	26	27	28
29	30	31				

APRIL
M	T	W	T	F	S	S
			1	2	3	4
5	6	7	8	9	10	11
12	13	14	15	16	17	18
19	20	21	22	23	24	25
26	27	28	29	30		

SEPTEMBER 2025

MONDAY	TUESDAY	WEDNESDAY	THURSDAY
1 Labor Day	2	3	4
8	9	10	11
15	16	17	18
22 First Day of Fall Rosh Hashanah Begins	23	24	25
29 ◑	30		

FRIDAY	SATURDAY	SUNDAY
5	6	7 ○
12	13	14 ◑
19	20	21 ●
26	27	28

LIVE WELL

Make a Fall "Wellness List." Autumn starts on September 22, so make a bucket list focused on your well-being. It's an excellent time for outdoor activities like hiking and leaf peeping, and seasonal produce will be at its peak. If you're affected by winter's short days, make the most of the current daylight while it lasts.

AUGUST

M	T	W	T	F	S	S
				1	2	3
4	5	6	7	8	9	10
11	12	13	14	15	16	17
18	19	20	21	22	23	24
25	26	27	28	29	30	31

OCTOBER

M	T	W	T	F	S	S
		1	2	3	4	5
6	7	8	9	10	11	12
13	14	15	16	17	18	19
20	21	22	23	24	25	26
27	28	29	30	31		

OCTOBER 2025

MONDAY	TUESDAY	WEDNESDAY	THURSDAY
		1 Yom Kippur Begins	**2**
6	**7** ○	**8**	**9**
13 Indigenous Peoples' Day ◑	**14**	**15**	**16**
20 Diwali Begins	**21** ●	**22**	**23**
27	**28**	**29** ◑	**30**

FRIDAY	SATURDAY	SUNDAY
3	4	5
10	11	12
17	18	19
24	25	26
31 Halloween		

LIVE WELL

Try an Indoor Plant. It might be nearing the end of outdoor gardening season, but you can still reap the feel-good benefits by adding some greenery to your home. If you have trouble keeping things alive, see if your thumb is any greener with low-maintenance picks like aloe vera and snake plants (they can tolerate your occasionally forgetting to water them).

SEPTEMBER

M	T	W	T	F	S	S
1	2	3	4	5	6	7
8	9	10	11	12	13	14
15	16	17	18	19	20	21
22	23	24	25	26	27	28
29	30					

NOVEMBER

M	T	W	T	F	S	S
					1	2
3	4	5	6	7	8	9
10	11	12	13	14	15	16
17	18	19	20	21	22	23
24	25	26	27	28	29	30

NOVEMBER 2025

MONDAY	TUESDAY	WEDNESDAY	THURSDAY
3	4	5 ○	6
10	11 Veterans Day	12 ◑	13
17	18	19	20 ●
24	25	26	27 Thanksgiving

FRIDAY	SATURDAY	SUNDAY
	1 All Saints' Day	**2** Daylight Saving Time Ends
7	**8**	**9**
14	**15**	**16**
21	**22**	**23**
28 ☽	**29**	**30** First Day of Advent

LIVE WELL

Have a "Me Day."
As the holiday season kicks off, don't forget to make room in your calendar for some personal activities you'll find restorative. Schedule a bonus day for yourself and plan activities that are good for you and make you feel energetic or happy. Cook a healthy recipe you've had your eye on, start a puzzle while sipping a cup of tea, buy yourself a new book, or take a workout class you've been trying to find time for.

OCTOBER

M	T	W	T	F	S	S
		1	2	3	4	5
6	7	8	9	10	11	12
13	14	15	16	17	18	19
20	21	22	23	24	25	26
27	28	29	30	31		

DECEMBER

M	T	W	T	F	S	S
1	2	3	4	5	6	7
8	9	10	11	12	13	14
15	16	17	18	19	20	21
22	23	24	25	26	27	28
29	30	31				

DECEMBER 2025

MONDAY	TUESDAY	WEDNESDAY	THURSDAY
1	2	3	4 ○
8	9	10	11 ◑
15	16	17	18
22	23	24 Christmas Eve	25 Christmas Day
29	30	31 New Year's Eve	

FRIDAY	SATURDAY	SUNDAY
5	6	7
12	13	14 Hanukkah Begins
19	20 ●	21 First Day of Winter
26 Kwanzaa Begins	27 ◗	28

LIVE WELL

Be Generous.
Research reveals that giving gifts prompts the flow of feel-good brain chemicals. If you consider yourself crafty, you can double down on that joyful vibe by creating something homemade this holiday season. DIY projects may help lower stress and increase happiness, studies show.

NOVEMBER

M	T	W	T	F	S	S
					1	2
3	4	5	6	7	8	9
10	11	12	13	14	15	16
17	18	19	20	21	22	23
24	25	26	27	28	29	30

JANUARY

M	T	W	T	F	S	S
			1	2	3	4
5	6	7	8	9	10	11
12	13	14	15	16	17	18
19	20	21	22	23	24	25
26	27	28	29	30	31	

FIND YOUR CALM

Welcome to the year of powerful, positive changes! This planner can help you get a handle on one of the biggest challenges we all face—everyday stress—and find new ways to restore a sense of calm, which is important for better health.

While stress may seem like a tricky topic to tackle, in reality stress is simply a natural reaction to perceived threats—in fact, sometimes feeling that stress can help you overcome tough situations like a looming work deadline or a spat with a friend. But when stress becomes normal, we can't always see what it's doing to our physical and mental health. Finding the right balance is key.

Each season we'll focus on a different health priority, with week-to-week advice for making small shifts in your daily routine that, over time, can make a lasting difference. Plus, you'll find a special section that shows you how to tap into the power of your own intuition and keep track of the advice you receive from your medical team. Here's to better health and more peace!

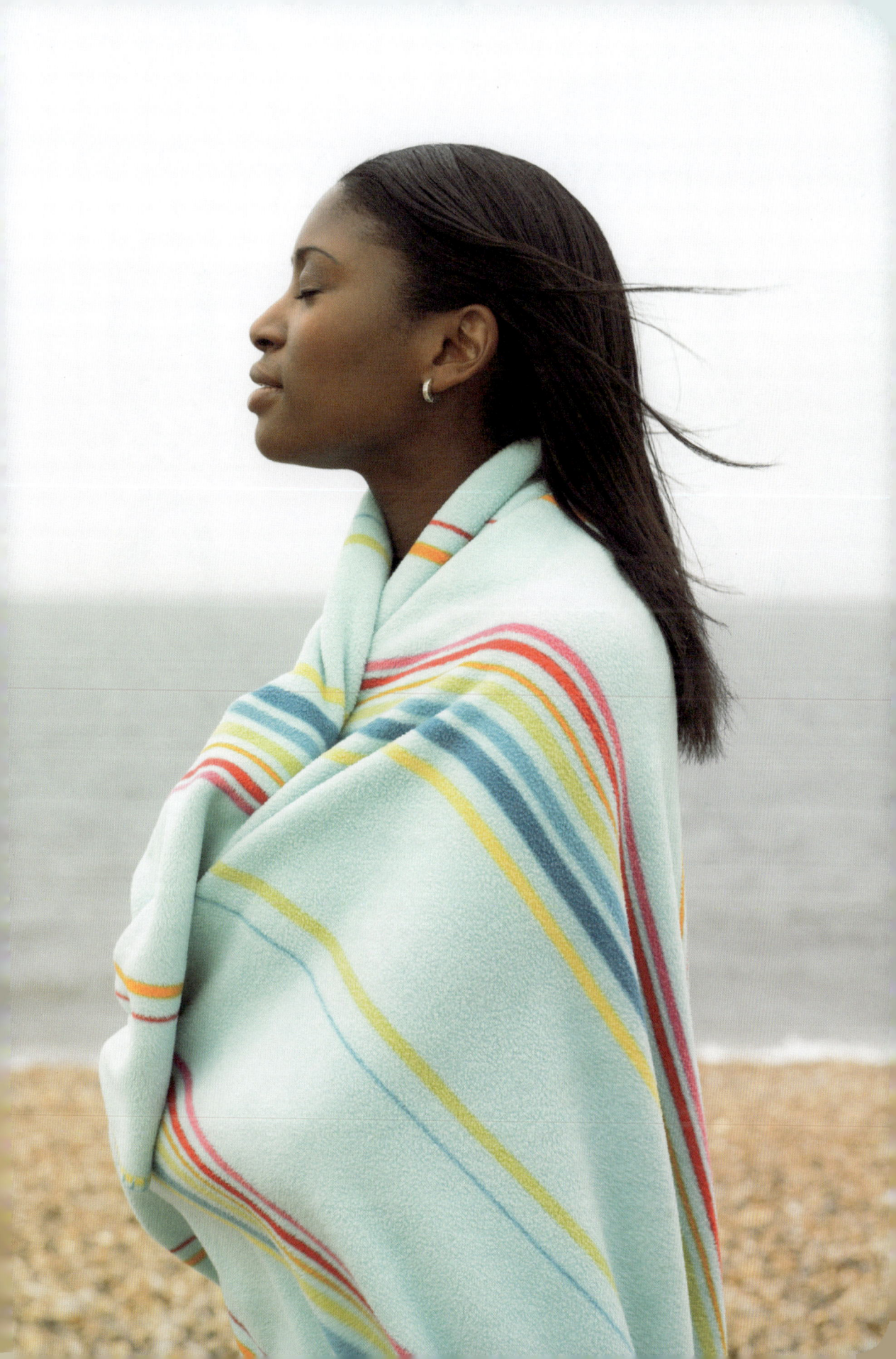

How Are You?

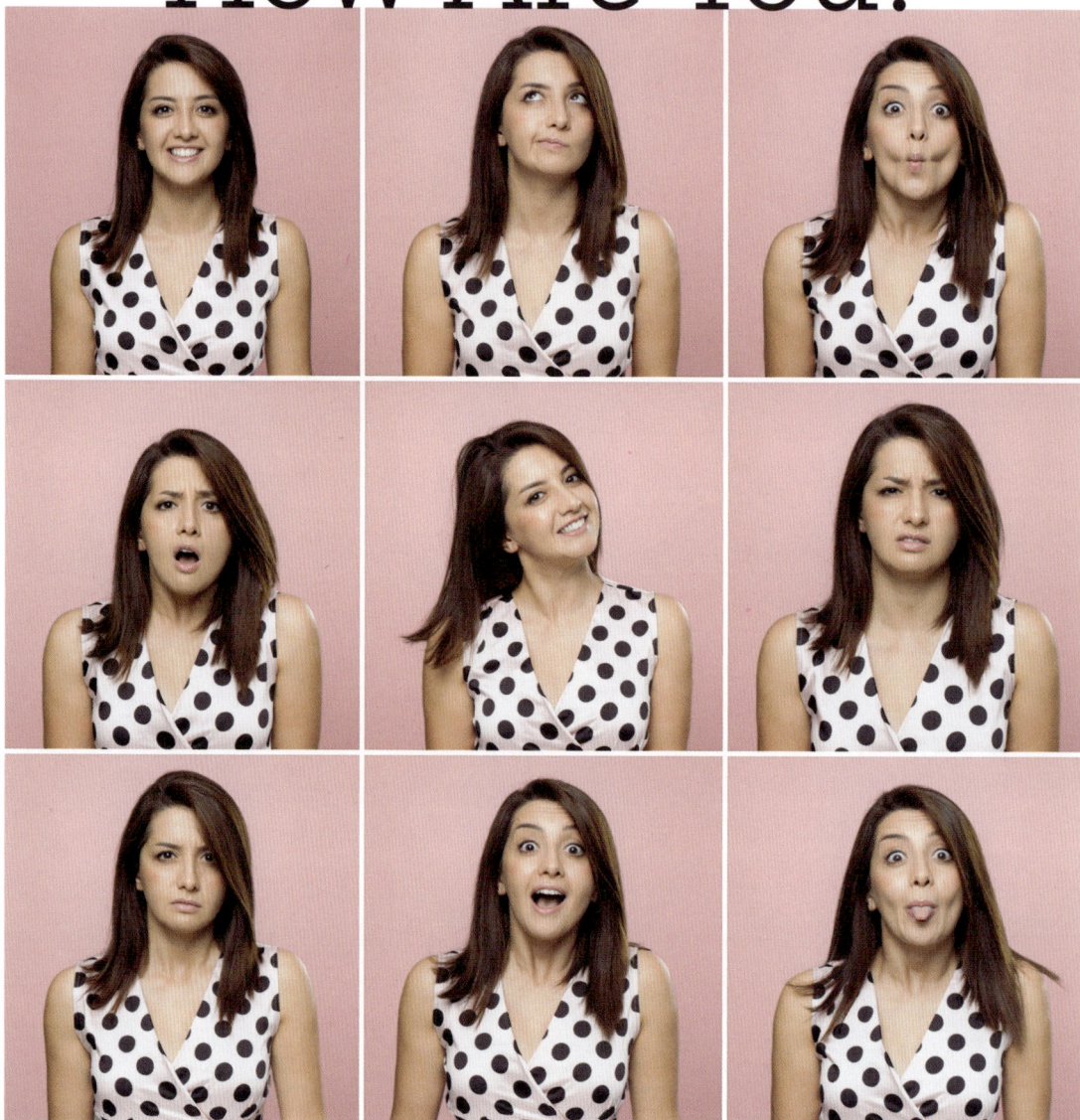

LET'S start by taking a moment to be emotionally honest. Chances are your answer to this question is "OK, I guess," "Blah," or—most likely—"Hmm, I don't know." Most of us ignore our emotions unless they are absolutely screaming. The chatter of our busy brains or the distraction of an endless to-do list often drowns out our feelings. When we do tune in to them, we may struggle to put into words how we feel or judge ourselves harshly for having the "wrong" emotions ("I'm so petty to feel envious of my best friend!").

Adding to the confusion: The current culture of toxic positivity (Good vibes only!) views some of our emotions as unacceptable. Grief, regret, and disappointment are seen as signs that something is wrong and needs fixing, unnecessary detours along our rightful path to constant joy. "There is pressure to think, *I have so much to feel grateful for—I don't have the right to be sad*," says therapist Whitney Goodman, author of *Toxic Positivity: Keeping It Real in a World Obsessed with Being Happy.* "But denying your feelings creates inner turmoil and shame that keeps you stuck."

In fact, all of our emotions—the good, the bad, and the ugly—can be powerful sources of wisdom and insight if we learn to attend to them. A new field of research into "emodiversity" has led to intriguing insights. For example, a groundbreaking study of more than 37,000 participants found that people who reported experiencing a wide variety of emotions in their daily lives were physically and mentally healthier compared with those who could cite only a few feelings.

Take a moment right now to check in with yourself. "Emotions are messengers. Even the ones that we don't like are trying to let us know something about what we need. If we ignore those messages, it will impact our relationships, our sleep, and our productivity," explains Charryse Johnson, Ph.D., LCMHC, founder of Jade Integrative Counseling and Wellness in Charlotte, NC.

The good news is that understanding and managing our feelings are skills we can all get better at. Emotions come in as many shades as an enormous pile of crayons, and they give life its vivid richness.

Having Mixed Emotions Is Totally Normal

Though they rarely make Instagram highlight reels, uncomfortable feelings are often part of even happy times like vacations, holidays, and graduations. Simply acknowledging this tension can help defuse it. For example, weddings are full of joy and celebration, but other emotions—sadness, exhaustion, anxiety—are likely part of the picture too.

Understanding that it's natural to have a mix of feelings even on "happy" occasions means you won't be blindsided or declare the experience totally ruined when you have a negative emotion. That will make you more open to the positives as well.

Contemplate a big event in your life. What mix of emotions did you experience? Was one feeling bigger than the others during this important time? Mentally divide the pie chart below to represent your mixed feelings.

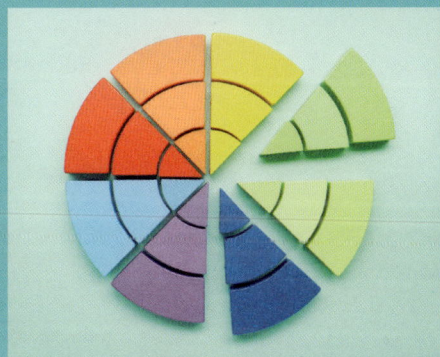

Give Your Mood a Boost

LET'S BE REAL: Nobody is perfectly happy 100% of the time. Just as life has its ups and downs, our mental states do too. "We're emotional beings, so mood changes throughout the day and our lives are normal," says Rachel Goldman, Ph.D., a psychologist and clinical assistant professor in the department of psychiatry at NYU Grossman School of Medicine. "Many things can impact our mood."

Various situations, interactions with others, and our jobs are common mood influencers; lifestyle factors like how well we sleep and what we eat also play a role.

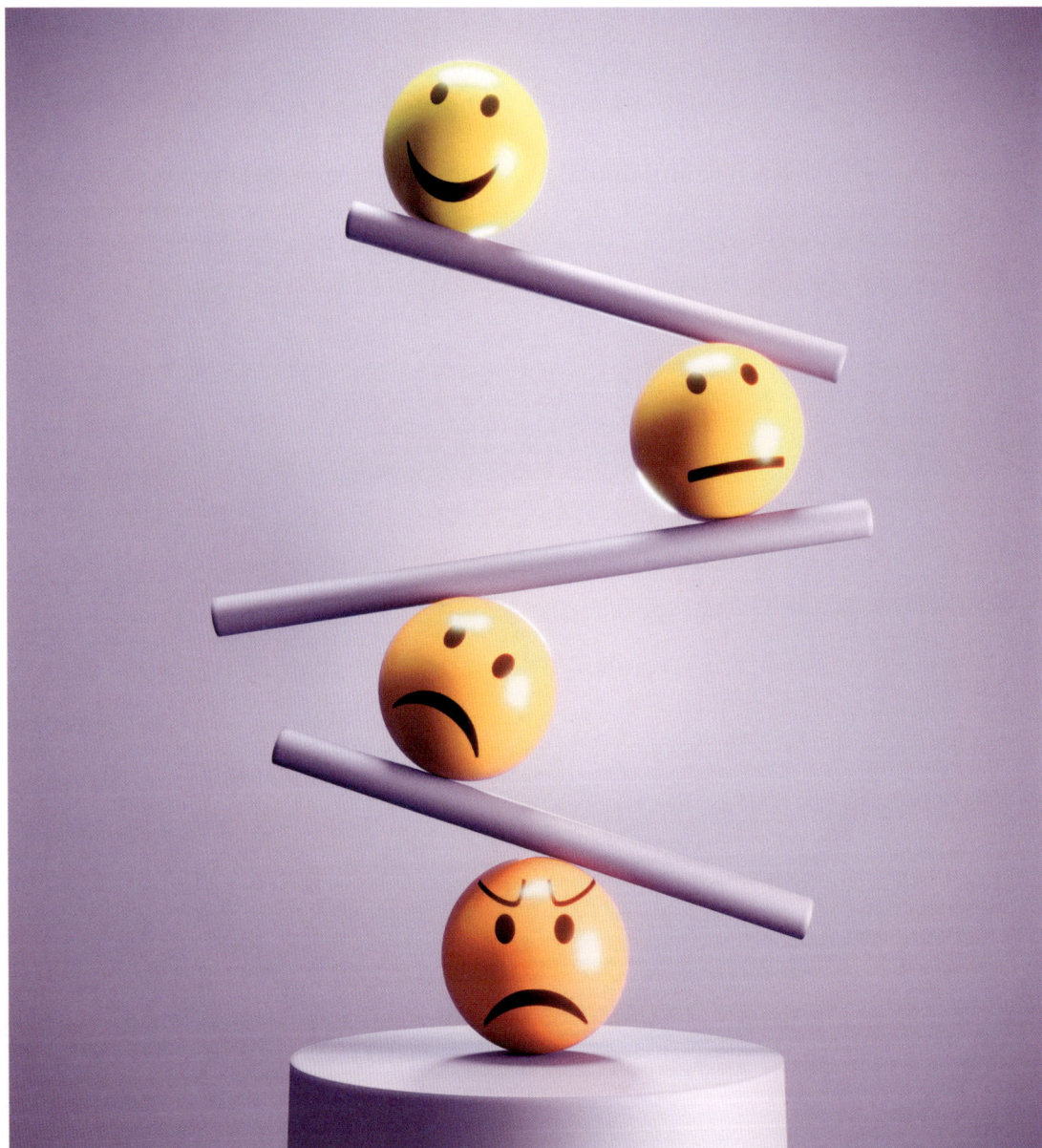

One-off bad days are a drain, but they aren't too worrisome. Being consistently stuck on a mood roller coaster, though, can affect your physical health if you don't find a way to get off of it.

"The mind-body connection is real. Our bodies respond to the way we feel, think, and act," says Goldman, so feeling chronically off-kilter mentally can trigger issues that are tied to disease risks such as high blood pressure and inflammation. That's why one of the most powerful skills you can master is turning your mood around—and you don't need much spare time to feel a change! Next time you're feeling a little low, try one of these almost instant mood flippers from Judy Ho, Ph.D., a neuropsychologist and the author of *Stop Self-Sabotage: Six Steps to Unlock Your True Motivation.*

IF YOU HAVE ONE MINUTE: Think of three things you're grateful for right now, big or small. "When you acknowledge the positives, it contributes to how you feel. It's based in cognitive behavioral therapy, and the thought shift can result in an instantaneous mood shift," Ho says.

✿ **SUPERCHARGE IT** and speak your thoughts out loud. "You can amplify the feeling of gratitude by hearing those thoughts articulated to yourself and those around you," says Ho.

IF YOU HAVE 5 MINUTES: Revisit a pleasant memory, whether it's recent or from long ago. "This is based on narrative therapy, in which you use stories of your life to enhance your mood," says Ho. Remembering how you felt in those moments can lift your spirits by bringing on similar emotions.

✿ **SUPERCHARGE IT** and look at a photo or video tied to that memory. "Really paint a vivid picture and engage your five senses—what did you see, hear, feel, smell, etc.? Tap into as much detail as possible and savor the experience," Ho suggests.

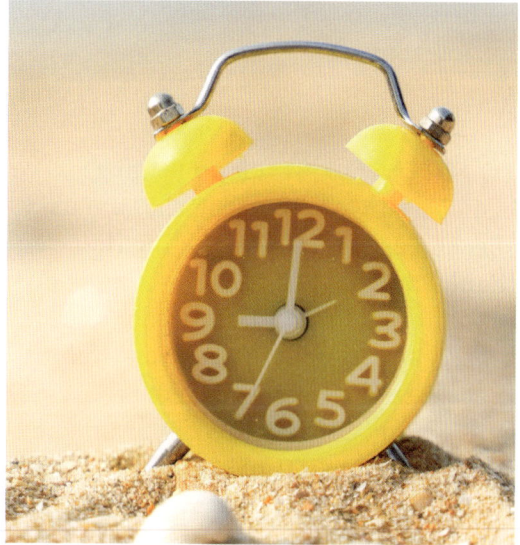

IF YOU HAVE 10 MINUTES: Create a joy list. Says Ho, "Set a timer and write down whatever happiness-inducing things come to mind. Don't edit yourself. It's OK to include grand items (a vacation to Bali!) as well as small things like the taste of morning coffee. When you're in a negative headspace, it can be hard to think of positives, so things that are quick and visceral and that engage the senses are helpful activities to put on the list."

✿ **SUPERCHARGE IT** and commit to doing something on that list within the next 24 hours. After you complete it, rate your level of enjoyment and mood on a scale from 1 to 5. "This lets you know what's working and what's not," says Ho. "Eventually, the goal is to do something on your joy list that you've rated a 3 or higher every day."

Embrace Tranquility

Managing stress and anxiety is only half the battle. There are also some tried-and-true ways to improve your sense of control over whatever may be bothering you at the moment. Consider the following:

CROSS SOMETHING SIMPLE OFF YOUR TO-DO LIST.
Pick one thing you've been putting off—making that annual checkup appointment, sending that thank-you note to a friend—and just do it. Chores like this take up space in our brain, causing underlying stress. Taking even one of them off your mental list will give you a sense of accomplishment and a few moments of "Aah..."

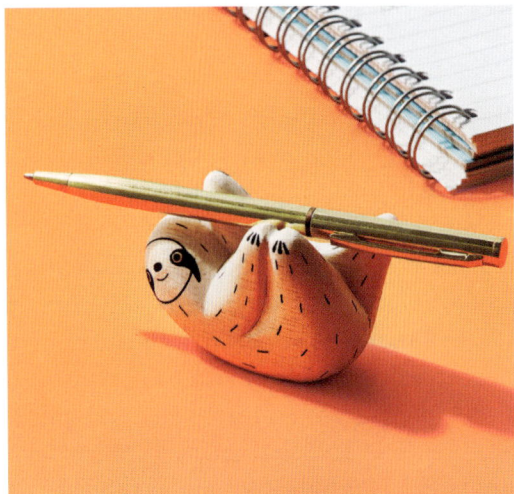

PLAY YOUR FAVORITE SONG.
Numerous studies have demonstrated that listening to music helps reduce stress, and that listening to music with the intention of relaxing helps lower cortisol levels. Also, choosing an energizing tune can make you feel more alert and focused.

STRETCH OUT.
Stretching relaxes and loosens your body, of course, but there's also evidence that it can ease your mind. One study showed that 10 minutes of stretching slowly and mindfully could reduce anxiety. So do some downward-facing dog poses, breathe in and out deeply, and let the de-stressing begin.

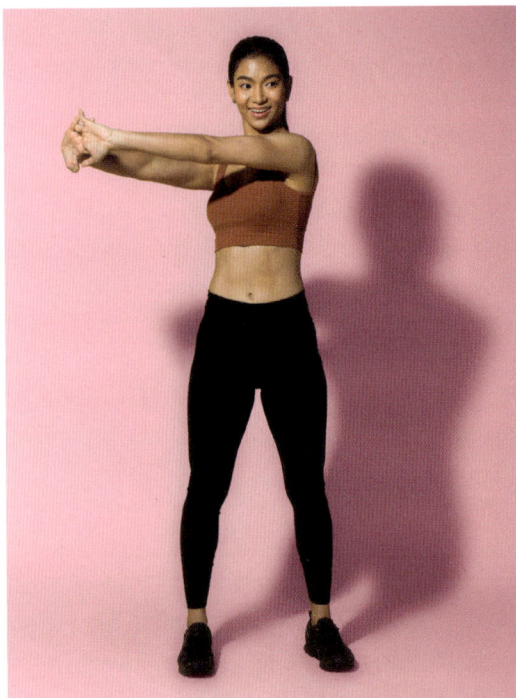

USE THE 3-3-3 RULE.
Many therapists and psychologists recommend using this grounding technique to help alleviate anxiety in the moment: Look around and name three things you can see, then identify three things you can feel, and finally, move three parts of your body. This redirects your attention from spiraling anxious thoughts to very specific tasks that center your thinking and calm you down.

GIVE YOUR FACE A COLD PLUNGE.
Splashing ice-cold water on your face for 15 to 20 seconds won't just wake you up—there's evidence that it also engages your body's relaxation system to counter-act your stress response. An option that is more makeup friendly: Hold an ice cube or a chilly drink against your skin. The sensory experience can quickly distract you from worrying thoughts.

HAVE A LAUGH. Cackling at something hilarious can be downright therapeutic: Studies indicate that laughing at a funny YouTube video has a significant effect on perceived stress. Laughter has been shown to reduce stress, anxiety, and depression by suppressing hormones like cortisol. Also, it stimulates circulation and helps muscles relax, which may reduce physical symptoms of anxiety.

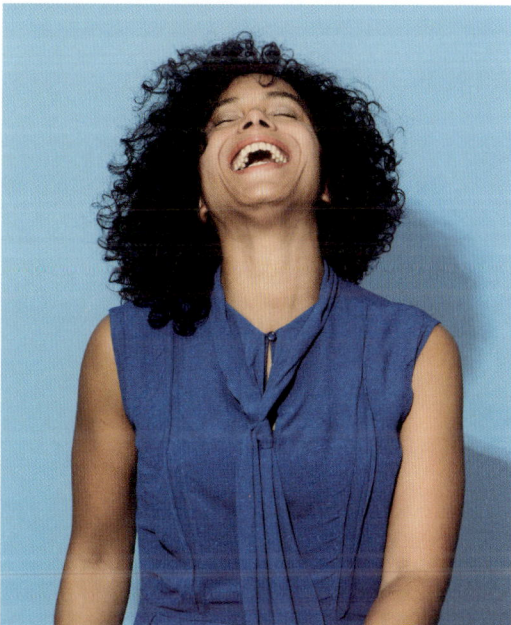

TAKE A WALK OUTSIDE. A brisk 10-minute stroll can lower anxiety, research shows. Any sort of exercise is thought to boost mood-regulating brain chemicals like serotonin, which helps induce calmness. And just being outside in fresh air has a relaxing effect on the mind.

DO SOME HEAVY PETTING. Playing with dogs and cats is good for both improving your mood and offering stress relief. Research also suggests that social interaction between people and their dogs increases levels of the feel-good hormone oxytocin. Any animal can be an emotional support animal.

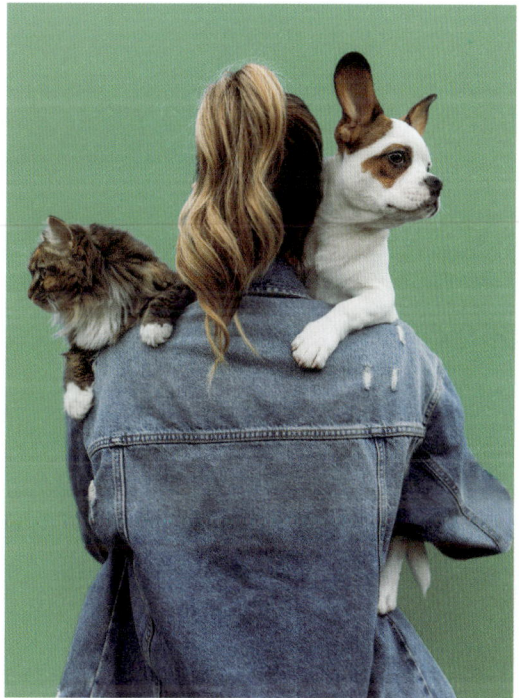

CANCEL SOMETHING. This one takes mere seconds! Look at your calendar and find one thing you really can skip, such as a social event you're not psyched about or a Zoom meeting that doesn't require your input. Politely bow out and replace it with... nothing! Your body and mind can rest and recharge.

YOUR PERSONAL
WELLNESS JOURNAL

When it comes to your health, it's critical to use every tool in your toolbox, including seemingly irrational feelings. So this year, while you're addressing your stress and restoring your calm, it makes sense to practice honing your intuition as well, and—perhaps just as important—to speak about it in a way that forces your health care team to pay attention. "When women are in tune with their bodies and feel empowered to share their insights with their physicians, that's when they should receive the best medical care," says Martha Gulati, M.D., a cardiologist at Cedars-Sinai Heart Institute in Los Angeles.

This section of your *Prevention Planner* is designed to help you do just that. You'll find a grid to keep track of all the different providers in your care team, as well as the medications and therapies they prescribe, so you keep all the practical details in one place. But there's something else you bring to the table that's just as important to share with your medical providers—your own firsthand hunch as to what might be wrong in the first place.

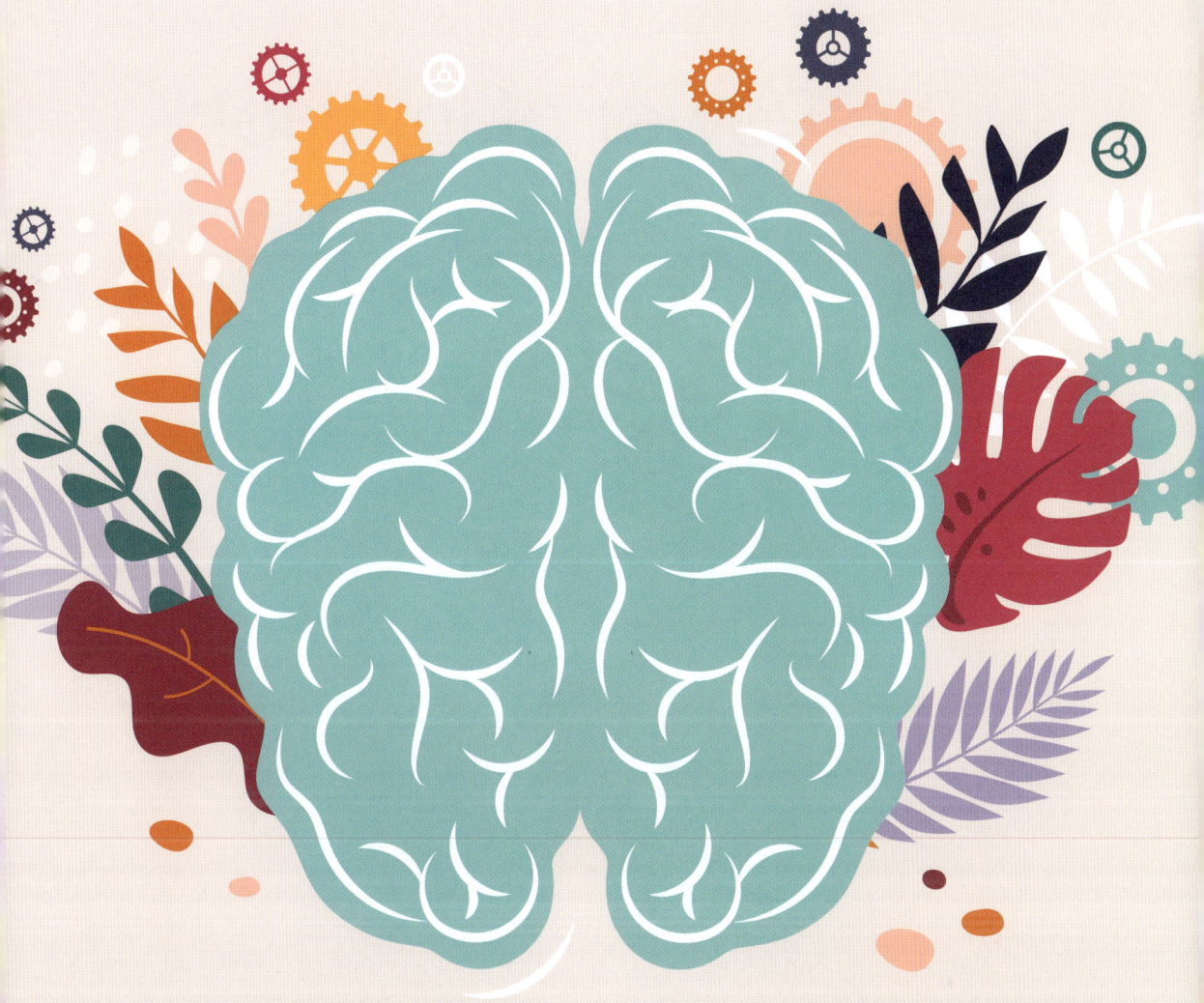

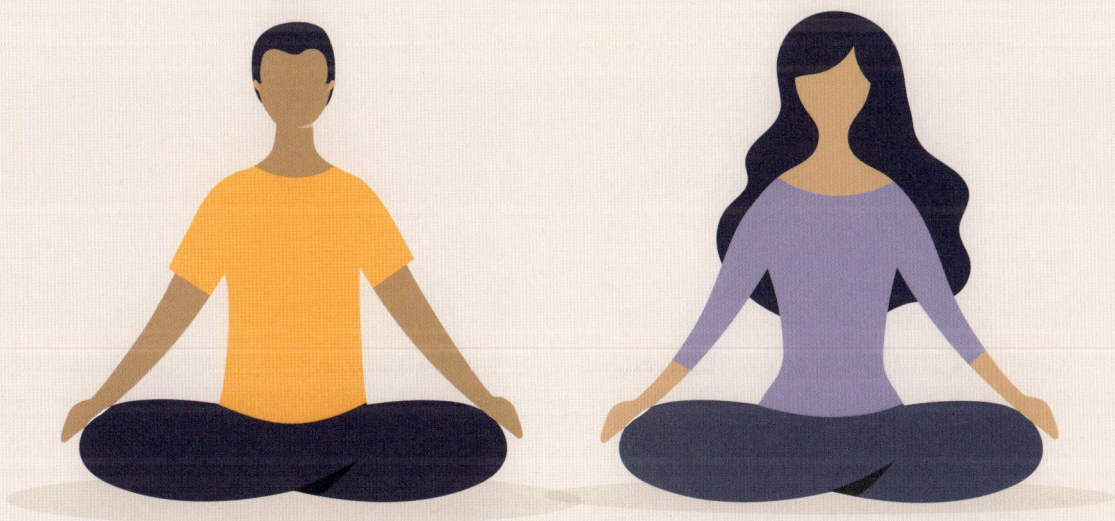

The Power of Intuition

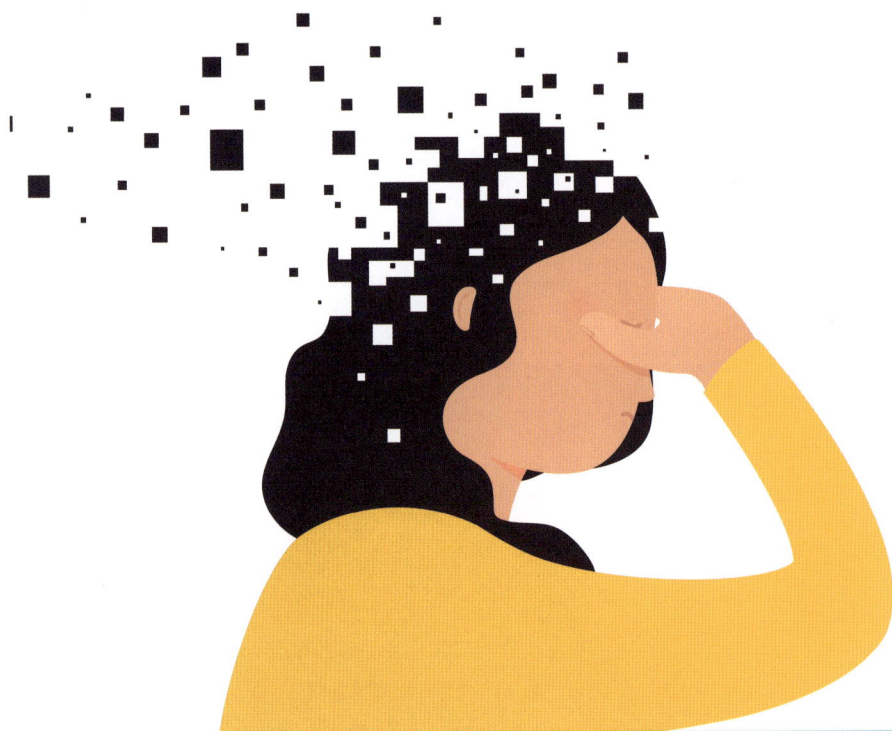

While advances in medicine have led to critically important diagnostic tools to identify and treat disease, we all have an underutilized symptom tracker operating in our subconscious mind. It's that sense you get that something doesn't feel right, when you notice a change in your body. It may be subtle, not even identifiable, but you know it's there—so when that internal system offers up an alert, it's a good idea to pay attention.

Of course, there are times when that signal is off—when you are convinced you have COVID only to get three negative test results in a row, or when what you are sure is appendicitis turns out to be just gas. Such errors often arise from a potent mix of anxiety about the fragility of life combined with information overload, with every Google search of a symptom taking you down a rabbit hole leading to potential diseases.

But there are times when that internal alert system can be a crucial tool: A pair of studies—one published in *BMC Primary Care* in 2022 and the other in the *British Journal of General Practice* in 2023—reported that primary care physicians found patients' instincts about their health to be a valuable part of clinical care. In another study, researchers reported that patients' gut feelings about having cancer could be reason enough to pursue more testing. Such instincts, the studies say, are often what initially lead patients to contact their doctors, voicing their internal knowing with statements like "Something isn't right," "This just feels wrong," and "I feel different from normal."

How to Hone Your Gut Instinct

Medical intuition is a muscle we can all strengthen. This requires acknowledging sometimes irrational emotional hunches and then synthesizing them with focused, rational, and discriminating cognitive analysis, says Helen Marlo, Ph.D., dean of the School of Psychology at Notre Dame de Namur University in Belmont, CA. Keep these tips in mind:

SEPARATE ANXIETY FROM ILLNESS. It's tempting to let Dr. Google fuel concerns, Marlo says. If your mind spins after you read up on symptoms online, it could be anxiety talking, not intuition. If you consistently think you have conditions it turns out you don't have, consider meeting with a qualified counselor to explore these thoughts and help you distinguish between anxiety and genuine bodily signals.

CHECK IN WITH YOUR BODY. Get to know what normal feels like. For example, make a point to check in with your body as part of your exercise routine, asking yourself, How are my feet doing? How are my ankles doing? How are my knees? My heart? "When you tune in to your body regularly, you're better equipped to detect it when something feels off, says Marlo.

KEEP TRACK OF CHANGES. If you sense that something is different, pay attention: Track changes in this journal or snap a quick photo or video on your phone. That way, when you present a doctor with concerns, you'll have solid info to back up what you're feeling.

DON'T DISCOUNT DATA. Hard facts—things like family history, inconclusive lab studies, and even erratic smartwatch data—can help you assess a seemingly irrational hunch. Sometimes the data provides the push you need to support getting further testing or a second opinion even when your constellation of symptoms don't fit a particular algorithm.

BE BOLD. It's important to advocate for yourself, especially if you're a woman. Speak up, ask questions, and don't be scared to offend your doctor, says Dr. Gulati. You deserve a clear explanation of why something isn't a concern or why follow-up testing isn't necessary. Your health is worth having an uncomfortable conversation.

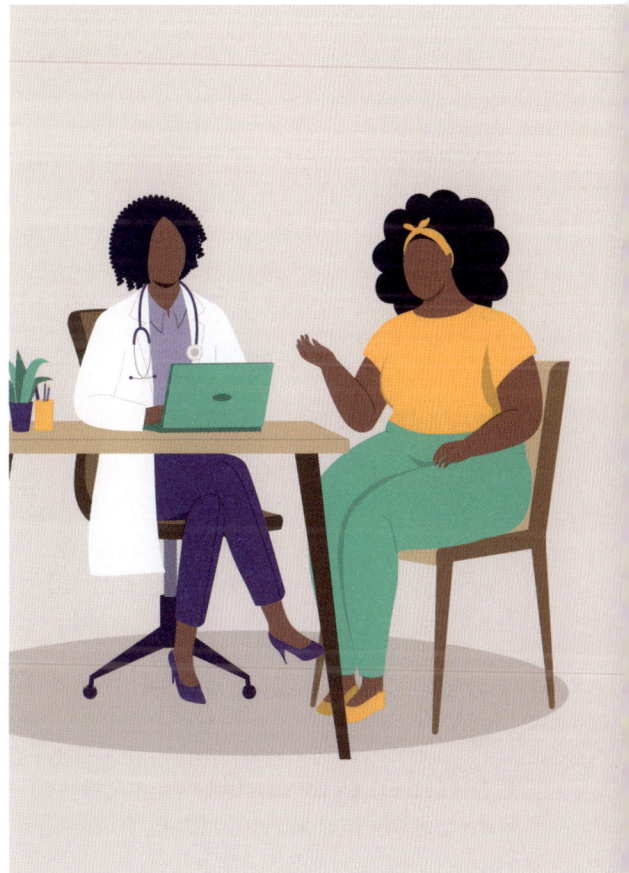

How to Face Your Health Fears

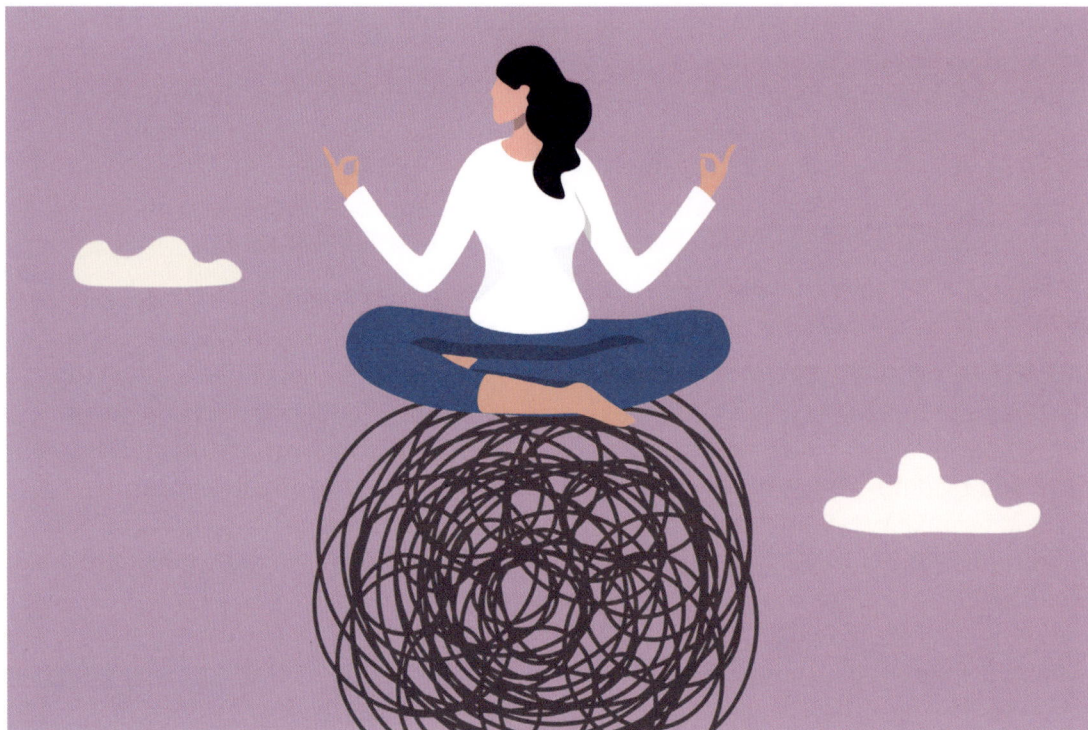

Developing a more realistic view of your health risks isn't easy. But a clear-eyed approach can bolster disease prevention by helping you focus on what matters, says Rebecca Hubbard, Ph.D., a licensed clinical psychologist based in Chicago who specializes in wellness and mental health. Try these strategies.

NURTURE YOUR EMOTIONAL SIDE.
Leaning on friends or faith can help you grapple with uncertainties. "Religion can have a positive impact on our health because it helps us tolerate the uncontrollable a bit better," Hubbard says. Therapy is effective for severe anxiety related to health, she adds.

CONSIDER EVERYTHING that affects your well-being. Start by identifying the things you can control, such as your behavior and the screenings you get, and those you can't control, like your age and your DNA. "It's scary to acknowledge the parts we're not in control of," Hubbard says. "But you don't have to do it alone."

LOOK AT THE FACTS OBJECTIVELY.
"Our fear of cancer is out of date," argues David Ropeik, author of the book *Curing Cancerphobia: How Risk, Fear, and Worry Mislead Us.* "We still believe most cancer kills, and that's not true." In fact, many cancers are now treatable or curable—remembering that may make testing less frightening. Plus, some cancers, including some breast, prostate, and thyroid cancers, may never cause symptoms, so getting screened could help you feel empowered to spot problems.

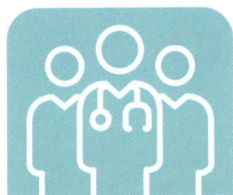

Your Health Care Team

Your primary care physician is best qualified to advise you on what best suits your health needs. For referrals to specialists, you can use this chart to keep all the details in one place.

SPECIALIST	CONTACT INFORMATION	SCHEDULED
PRIMARY CARE PHYSICIAN **Routine Tests:** Blood pressure, cholesterol and blood sugar screenings and referral for routine colonoscopy after age 45 **Frequency:** Annual	Name: _____ Address: _____ _____ Phone: _____	Date: Time:
DENTIST **Routine Tests:** X-rays to identify potential cavities, routine cleaning **Frequency:** Biannual	Name: _____ Address: _____ _____ Phone: _____	Date: Time:
GYNECOLOGIST **Routine Tests:** Pelvic exam and pap smear **Frequency:** Annual	Name: _____ Address: _____ _____ Phone: _____	Date: Time:
OPTOMETRIST **Routine Tests:** Eye exam and glaucoma screening **Frequency:** Every 2 years for people starting at age 40; annual after 65	Name: _____ Address: _____ _____ Phone: _____	Date: Time:
DERMATOLOGIST **Routine Tests:** Skin cancer screening **Frequency:** Annual unless advised otherwise	Name: _____ Address: _____ _____ Phone: _____	Date: Time:
OTHER	Name: _____ Address: _____ _____ Phone: _____	Date: Time:
OTHER	Name: _____ Address: _____ _____ Phone: _____	Date: Time:

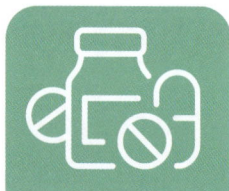

Your Medication Log

If your daily routine includes a variety of supplements and prescriptions, use this page to make it easier to keep track of what you need to take—as well as how much and when.

MORNING

TIME	MEDICATION	DOSAGE	WITH MEALS?
			Yes No
			Yes No
			Yes No
			Yes No

AFTERNOON

TIME	MEDICATION	DOSAGE	WITH MEALS?
			Yes No
			Yes No
			Yes No
			Yes No

EVENING

TIME	MEDICATION	DOSAGE	WITH MEALS?
			Yes No
			Yes No
			Yes No
			Yes No

SIDE EFFECTS

MEDICATION	WHAT TO WATCH FOR	WHAT I'VE EXPERIENCED

VISIT LOG

SAMPLE...

DOCTOR Amanda Jones   **DATE** 3/5/25   **TIME** 3:15

ISSUES I'M HAVING

My knee hurts when I squat or do steps. I always have to hold the railing to feel safe. Sometimes it aches at night.

BEFORE VISIT

WHAT I'VE TRIED/QUESTIONS TO ASK

I've tried icing it and I take Tylenol almost every day.

DOCTOR'S RECOMMENDATION

The doctor is referring me to an orthopedist for some more tests... x-rays and possibly an MRI.

AFTER VISIT

MY ACTION PLAN

Continue icing and try ibuprofen instead of Tylenol. Get the appointment scheduled with the orthopedist.

DOCTOR   **DATE**   **TIME**

ISSUES I'M HAVING

WHAT I'VE TRIED/QUESTIONS TO ASK

BEFORE VISIT

DOCTOR'S RECOMMENDATION

MY ACTION PLAN

AFTER VISIT

WELLNESS JOURNAL: VISIT LOG

DOCTOR

DATE

TIME

ISSUES I'M HAVING	WHAT I'VE TRIED/QUESTIONS TO ASK

BEFORE VISIT

DOCTOR'S RECOMMENDATION	MY ACTION PLAN

AFTER VISIT

DOCTOR

DATE

TIME

ISSUES I'M HAVING	WHAT I'VE TRIED/QUESTIONS TO ASK

BEFORE VISIT

DOCTOR'S RECOMMENDATION	MY ACTION PLAN

AFTER VISIT

DOCTOR _____ **DATE** _____ **TIME** _____

ISSUES I'M HAVING	WHAT I'VE TRIED/QUESTIONS TO ASK

BEFORE VISIT

DOCTOR'S RECOMMENDATION	MY ACTION PLAN

AFTER VISIT

DOCTOR _____ **DATE** _____ **TIME** _____

ISSUES I'M HAVING	WHAT I'VE TRIED/QUESTIONS TO ASK

BEFORE VISIT

DOCTOR'S RECOMMENDATION	MY ACTION PLAN

AFTER VISIT

WELLNESS JOURNAL: VISIT LOG

DOCTOR

DATE

TIME

ISSUES I'M HAVING

WHAT I'VE TRIED/QUESTIONS TO ASK

BEFORE
VISIT

DOCTOR'S RECOMMENDATION

MY ACTION PLAN

AFTER
VISIT

DOCTOR

DATE

TIME

ISSUES I'M HAVING

WHAT I'VE TRIED/QUESTIONS TO ASK

BEFORE
VISIT

DOCTOR'S RECOMMENDATION

MY ACTION PLAN

AFTER
VISIT

DOCTOR _____ **DATE** _____ **TIME** _____

ISSUES I'M HAVING	WHAT I'VE TRIED/QUESTIONS TO ASK

BEFORE VISIT

DOCTOR'S RECOMMENDATION	MY ACTION PLAN

AFTER VISIT

DOCTOR _____ **DATE** _____ **TIME** _____

ISSUES I'M HAVING	WHAT I'VE TRIED/QUESTIONS TO ASK

BEFORE VISIT

DOCTOR'S RECOMMENDATION	MY ACTION PLAN

AFTER VISIT

WELLNESS JOURNAL: VISIT LOG

DOCTOR _____ **DATE** _____ **TIME** _____

ISSUES I'M HAVING	WHAT I'VE TRIED/QUESTIONS TO ASK

BEFORE VISIT

DOCTOR'S RECOMMENDATION	MY ACTION PLAN

AFTER VISIT

DOCTOR _____ **DATE** _____ **TIME** _____

ISSUES I'M HAVING	WHAT I'VE TRIED/QUESTIONS TO ASK

BEFORE VISIT

DOCTOR'S RECOMMENDATION	MY ACTION PLAN

AFTER VISIT

DOCTOR _____ **DATE** _____ **TIME** _____

ISSUES I'M HAVING	WHAT I'VE TRIED/QUESTIONS TO ASK

BEFORE VISIT

DOCTOR'S RECOMMENDATION	MY ACTION PLAN

AFTER VISIT

DOCTOR _____ **DATE** _____ **TIME** _____

ISSUES I'M HAVING	WHAT I'VE TRIED/QUESTIONS TO ASK

BEFORE VISIT

DOCTOR'S RECOMMENDATION	MY ACTION PLAN

AFTER VISIT

WELLNESS JOURNAL: VISIT LOG

DOCTOR _____ **DATE** _____ **TIME** _____

ISSUES I'M HAVING	WHAT I'VE TRIED/QUESTIONS TO ASK

BEFORE VISIT

DOCTOR'S RECOMMENDATION	MY ACTION PLAN

AFTER VISIT

DOCTOR _____ **DATE** _____ **TIME** _____

ISSUES I'M HAVING	WHAT I'VE TRIED/QUESTIONS TO ASK

BEFORE VISIT

DOCTOR'S RECOMMENDATION	MY ACTION PLAN

AFTER VISIT

DOCTOR _____ **DATE** _____ **TIME** _____

ISSUES I'M HAVING	WHAT I'VE TRIED/QUESTIONS TO ASK

BEFORE VISIT

DOCTOR'S RECOMMENDATION	MY ACTION PLAN

AFTER VISIT

DOCTOR _____ **DATE** _____ **TIME** _____

ISSUES I'M HAVING	WHAT I'VE TRIED/QUESTIONS TO ASK

BEFORE VISIT

DOCTOR'S RECOMMENDATION	MY ACTION PLAN

AFTER VISIT

WINTER
EASE
YOUR MIND

We're all human, and we know there are some days when we feel really good and others when we get down in the dumps. And then there are times when our moods zip up and down! But learning how to keep things more steady, or at least more positive than negative, is a smart move for your health, both mental and physical. Becoming aware of your mood trends can help you get there.

"Mood awareness is an essential part of maintaining good mental health, and it doesn't mean you should feel positive all the time. In fact, that's an unrealistic expectation. Instead, try to be aware of what your mood is, what events or environments can trigger it, and learn ways to find balance," explains Himali Pandya, chief strategy and development officer at People USA, a mental health crisis prevention center in New York State. There are plenty of helpful calm-inducing strategies in this section, but let's start with figuring out how to name what you're feeling in the first place.

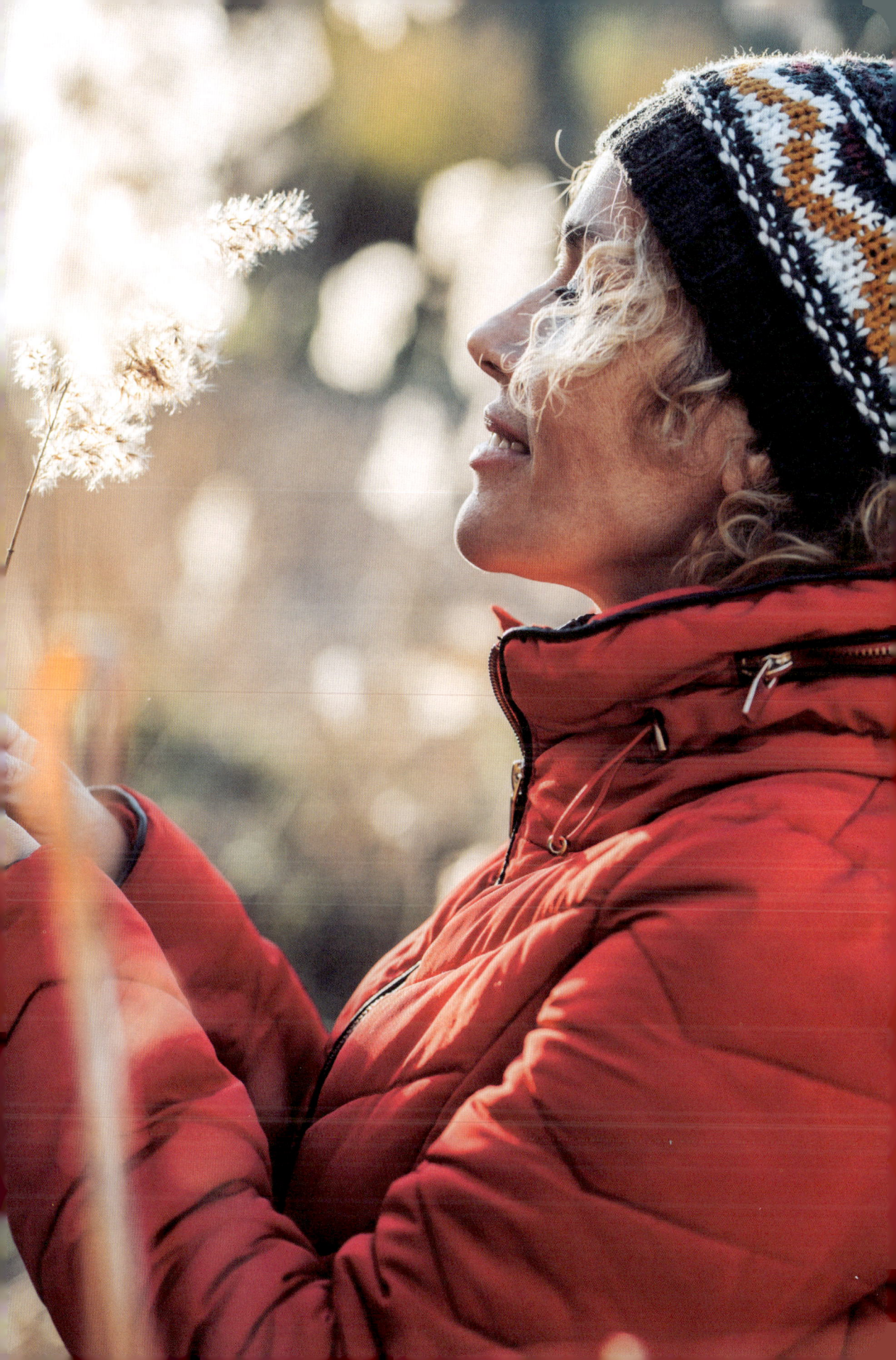

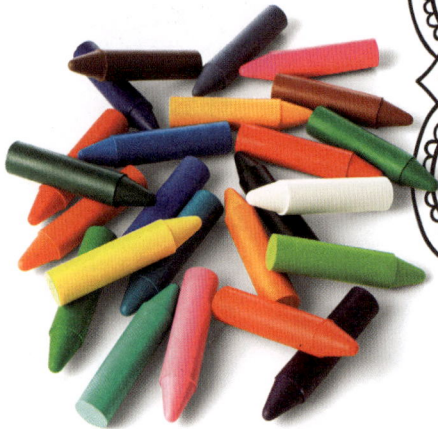

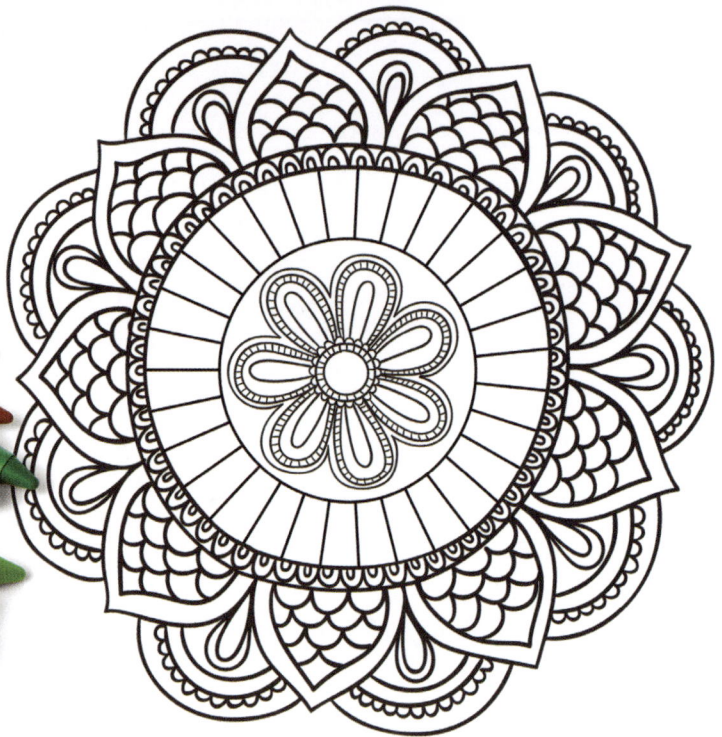

Mood Tracking for the Win

Getting a better handle on your emotional state throughout the day can be a powerful tool for understanding yourself and the range of feelings you likely experience. To start, try mood tracking. Below are three popular ways to do this; use one method per week, then think about which seemed to work best for you and consider building it into your routine going forward.

MOOD MANDALA. "People who are visual learners or who enjoy using colors to represent ideas and trends may find mood mandalas useful," says Pandya. These are graphic images you color according to how you're feeling. Assign a color to each of a handful of moods, then start in the middle of the image and spend a few minutes shading it in as your mood shifts throughout the day.

MOOD CHART. This is similar to journaling, but it offers a bit more structure that can help illuminate any patterns that seem to influence your mood status or mindset. Create a chart in your journal, on a whiteboard, or on a piece of paper, then draw columns for day of the week, mood, and mood-shifting factors. Make it fun by using colored pens or emoji stickers for tracking.

DAILY JOURNALING. Just let it flow! Each day, write down how you felt first thing in the morning, then at midday, and then in the evening. If you notice mindset changes between those time periods, jot those down too. It may also be helpful to write down anything that contributed to a shift in your mood throughout the day (such as dealing with a sick kid or having a fleeting positive or negative experience at work). "This is a great holistic wellness activity that can help you process daily experiences," says Pandya.

Breathe In Some Peace

One of the most powerful and scientifically proven stress-busting strategies is free, easy, and something that can be done anywhere: breathing. Taking a few deep, mindful breaths is an effective way to slow your heart rate and lower your blood pressure, and it can reduce anxiety within minutes. Being intentional is key, but don't get hung up on how-tos and counting if that puts you off. There's really no wrong way to do these techniques, so don't overthink it. Just sit comfortably and close your eyes, then try one of these three easy practices.

MINDFUL BREATHING. If you're a breathwork newbie, this one's for you. Just sit and do nothing but bring your attention to your breath for one minute. Surrender to this simplicity with the goal of working up to three minutes, suggests Roberto Benzo, M.D., director of the Mindful Breathing Lab at the Mayo Clinic in Rochester, MN.

✿ **HOW TO DO IT:** Set a timer for 60 seconds. If that's too long, start with 30 seconds. Inhale deeply and then exhale slowly and intentionally. If your mind wanders, focus on your breathing.

4-7-8 BREATHING. "This practice activates the body's relaxation response and reduces the release of stress hormones like cortisol," says Chiti Parikh, M.D., executive director of the Integrative Health and Wellbeing Program at Weill Cornell Medicine and New York-Presbyterian Hospital in New York City. She recommends doing 4-7-8 breathing before bedtime to help quiet your thoughts and make falling asleep easier.

✿ **HOW TO DO IT:** Inhale through your nose for a count of four. Hold your breath for a count of seven. Exhale through your mouth for a count of eight. Repeat this cycle at least three times.

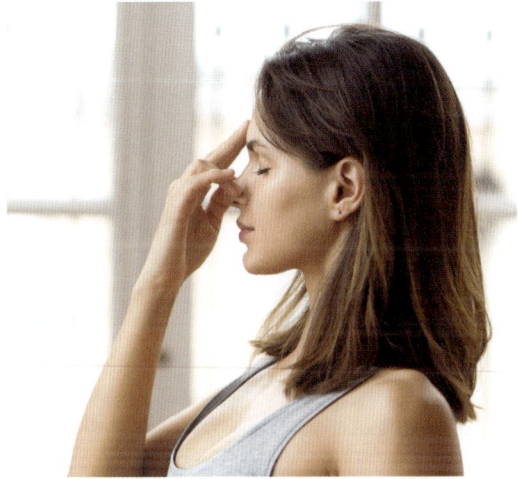

ALTERNATE-NOSTRIL BREATHING. Research shows that this yoga-based breathing exercise significantly reduces stress and improves lung function. The alternate-nostril action helps you stay focused on your breathing, which is usually on autopilot.

✿ **HOW TO DO IT:** Put your right thumb over your right nostril and inhale through your left nostril. Release that nostril, then place your ring finger over your left nostril and exhale via your right one. Without moving your finger, inhale through your right nostril, close it with your thumb, and exhale from your left one. Inhale through your left nostril, then close that nostril and exhale from your right one. Go back and forth like this for 11 rounds.

BELLY BREATHING. This is a simple yet powerful way to cater to your body and your mind. Breathing this way can lower blood pressure, decrease muscle tension, increase blood circulation, reduce GI symptoms, strengthen the pelvic floor, and quiet the mind to zap stress. Lindsey Benoit O'Connell, C.S.C.S., a meditation expert and founder of The LAB Wellness, teaches you to master this deep-breathing technique—follow along, then practice it at least a few times a week.

❀ **HOW TO DO IT:** Find a comfortable place to sit (or, to really target your pelvic region, lie down with your knees bent). Put one hand on your chest and the other on your abdomen just below your rib cage. Inhale through your nose for four to five seconds, filling your belly with air and focusing your attention on its rise. Hold for three seconds and tighten your abdomen. Then exhale slowly through your mouth for six seconds, releasing all the air.

Why Your Brain Needs to Snooze

Lack of sleep affects your ability to regulate your emotions, making handling daily stresses even harder. (And being super stressed in general can keep you up at night, continuing the miserable cycle.) Exactly why isn't clear, but part of the reason is that sleep lets the brain regroup. "Healthy sleep repairs adaptive processing, functional brain activity, [and] integrity of the medial prefrontal cortex-amygdala connections, and thus improves the capacity to regulate emotions as well as an individual's well-being," concluded one literature review in the journal *AIMS Neuroscience*.

Of course, trouble sleeping is both a cause and a symptom of depression, which means it can be hard to untangle the real issue and feel better. What's more, when someone improves their sleep it's more likely to wind up improving their mood than treating depression and hoping they start to sleep better, says Joseph M. Dzierzewski, Ph.D., vice president of research and scientific affairs at the National Sleep Foundation. After treatment for depression, he adds, "poor sleep is likely to be one of the remaining symptoms after your mood is improved."

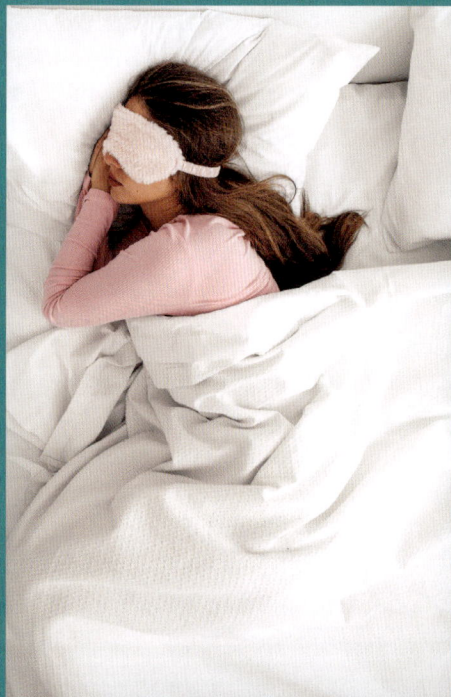

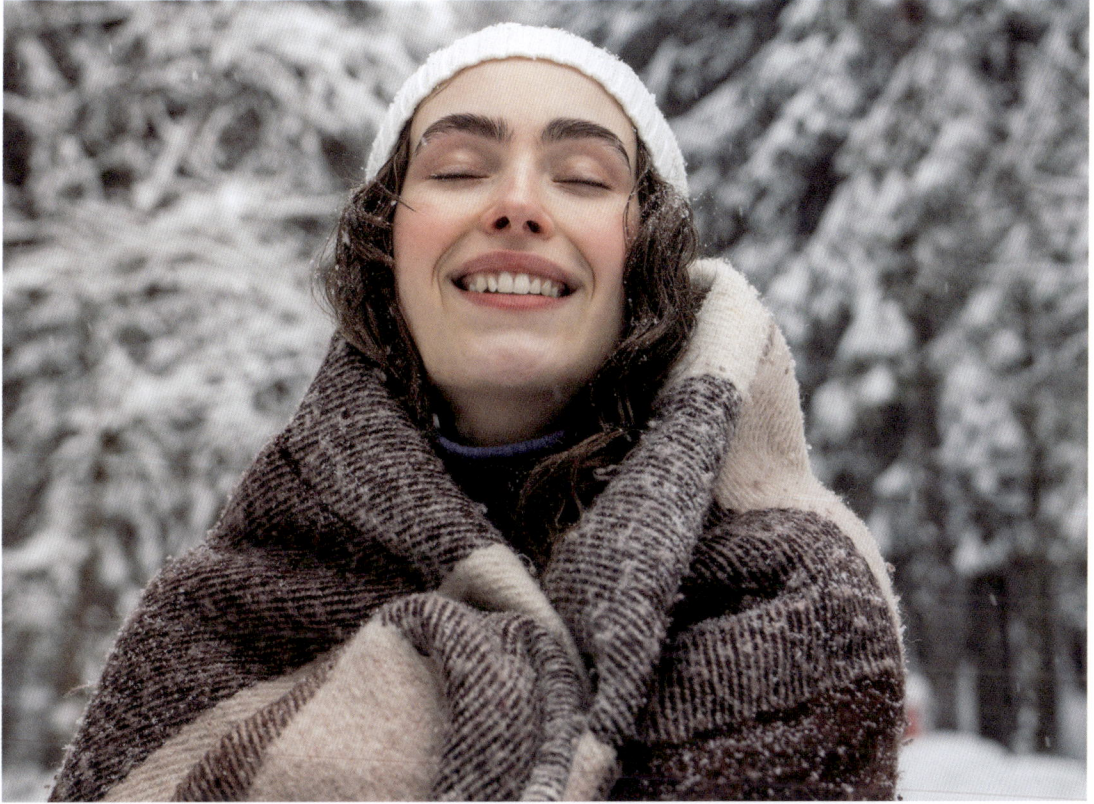

Take a Mental Health Day

Relaxing and recharging your mental/emotional batteries is crucial for keeping your nervous system from getting stuck in overdrive. When you need more than a quick stress fix, have a "me day." Judith Gulko, Ph.D., a psychologist in Coral Springs, FL, shares her prescription for using much-needed mental health time:

SOCIALIZE WITH OTHERS. Plan your day to coincide with a friend's. Get a joint massage, do karaoke together, or take a long walk while reminiscing about good times or planning some for the future.

OBSERVE YOUR STATE OF MIND. Whatever you choose to do (or not do), be chill. "Even yoga can be stressful if your perfectionism is triggered," Gulko says. Slow down and be present for every activity so you can return to work feeling truly recharged.

HAVE FUN. Dance around your living room or break out your kids' bubble blower or coloring books. Participating in playful activities—video games count!—has been found to lower adults' feelings of stress (along with their blood pressure). That's because play releases dopamine and other feel-good chemicals, research has found.

MAYBE DO NOTHING. If you're always on the go, the best way to spend this day might be to sleep in, then lounge around in your pj's daydreaming in the back yard or vegging out to mindless TV.

JANUARY 2026

MONDAY	TUESDAY	WEDNESDAY	THURSDAY
			1 New Year's Day
5	6	7	8
12	13	14	15
19 Martin Luther King Jr. Day	20	21	22
26 ◑	27	28	29

FRIDAY	SATURDAY	SUNDAY
2	3 ○	4
9	10 ◑	11
16	17	18 ●
23	24	25
30	31	

STRESS LESS

Light a Candle. If you're feeling the winter blues, filling the room with a favorite scent may offer the mood boost you need—and a candle that looks pretty or has a fun message may lift your spirits even more. You can find a variety of decorative candles featuring things wax roses, sprinkles and sequins, or just choose one with a quippy name such as "Be Kind to Your Mind."

DECEMBER

M	T	W	T	F	S	S
1	2	3	4	5	6	7
8	9	10	11	12	13	14
15	16	17	18	19	20	21
22	23	24	25	26	27	28
29	30	31				

FEBRUARY

M	T	W	T	F	S	S
						1
2	3	4	5	6	7	8
9	10	11	12	13	14	15
16	17	18	19	20	21	22
23	24	25	26	27	28	

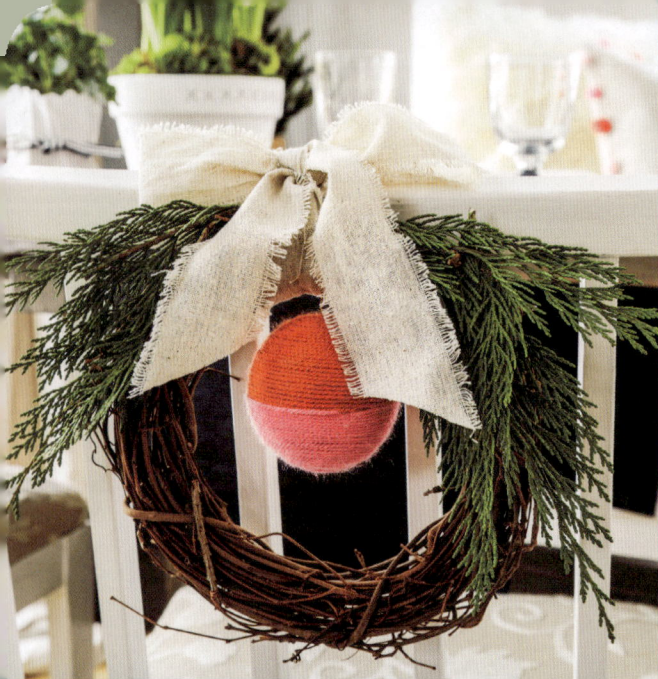

December 29– January 4

2025–2026

M	T	W	T	F	S	S
29	30	31	1	2	3	4
5	6	7	8	9	10	11
12	13	14	15	16	17	18
19	20	21	22	23	24	25
26	27	28	29	30	31	

ADD MORE JOY TO YOUR WINTER

Just as other mammals change their behavior in the winter, it makes sense for us to do so as well. But that doesn't mean hibernating like a bear until the trees bud again. Instead of mourning beach days and backyard barbecues, expand on the fun things you do only in winter. Take these steps to make your winter happier and less stressful.

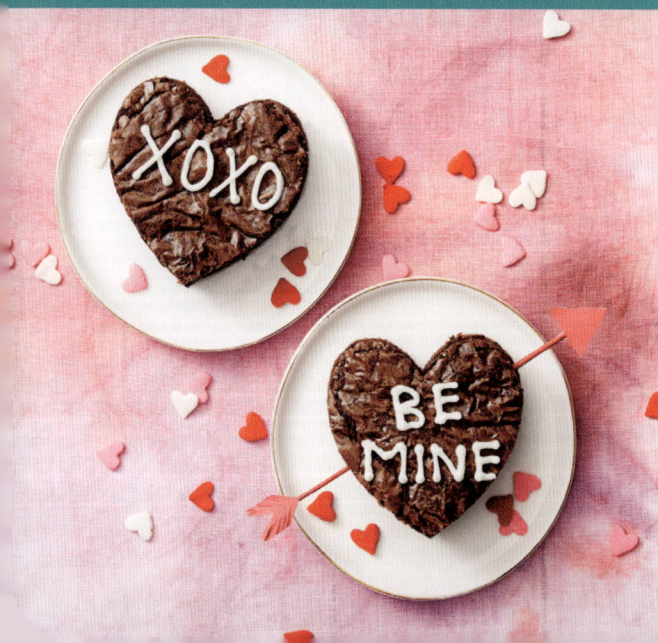

Try This Now

Think about your favorite holiday traditions. Maybe you love your family's annual latke party, or the Secret Santa gift exchange you've had for the past 30 years, or baking cookies for your coworkers, or decorating the house with childhood knickknacks. Brainstorm ways to carry some of those activities into January and February. "If you love Christmas baking, make Valentine's cookies," says Kari Leibowitz, Ph.D., a health psychologist and the author of How to Winter. "If you love all the socializing that happens around the holidays, host book club meetings, dinner parties, video game nights, or other gatherings after the holidays are over."

29 Monday

30 Tuesday

31 Wednesday

1 Thursday New Year's Day

2 Friday

3 Saturday ○

4 Sunday

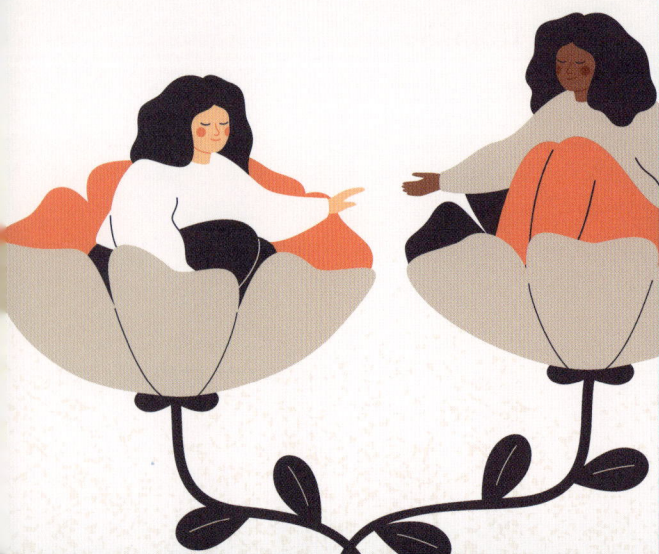

January
5–11
2026

M	T	W	T	F	S	S
			1	2	3	4
5	6	7	8	9	10	11
12	13	14	15	16	17	18
19	20	21	22	23	24	25
26	27	28	29	30	31	

MAKE NEW FRIENDS

You may have lots of friends, but if you're still feeling unsatisfied with your social life, it's never too late to form new bonds. Maybe you can strike up a conversation with someone you regularly see at the coffee shop or the dog park. It may feel uncomfortable at first because it involves the risk of rejection, but making new friends is possible.

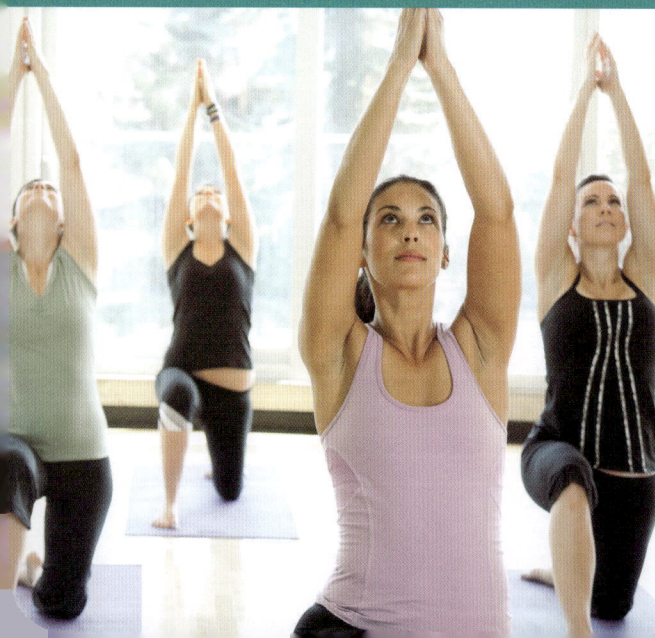

Here's What to Do

To start, look for natural connections. Groups such as pickleball leagues, cooking classes, and book clubs can introduce you to new people with similar interests. This can keep things from feeling awkward. "When you join a group, you're focused on an activity, so you'll have a safety net as you get to know people," says Tracy Brower, Ph.D., a sociologist and the author of *The Secrets to Happiness at Work*. And remember that friendship is about showing up. "If you go to yoga once, you're not going to connect, but if you keep showing up, you generate familiarity. Then it's easier to say, 'Let's go get a smoothie after class.'"

5 Monday

6 Tuesday

7 Wednesday

8 Thursday

9 Friday

10 Saturday ◑

11 Sunday

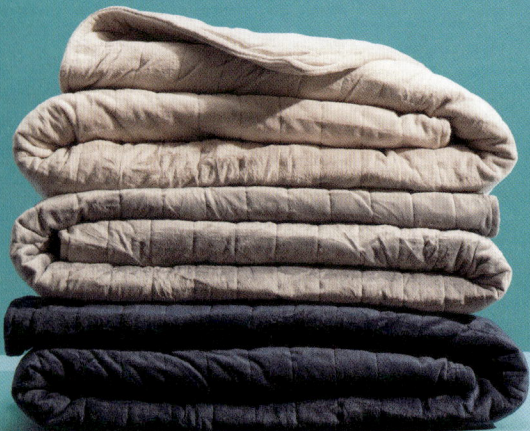

January
12–18
2026

M	T	W	T	F	S	S
			1	2	3	4
5	6	7	8	9	10	11
12	13	14	15	16	17	18
19	20	21	22	23	24	25
26	27	28	29	30	31	

TRY A WEIGHTED BLANKET

If you suffer from insomnia or anxiety, you know how frustrating it can be to lie awake in bed for hours on end. That's where a weighted blanket can come to the rescue: These blankets are typically filled with glass beads, with the added weight helping to create a relaxing feeling of being hugged.

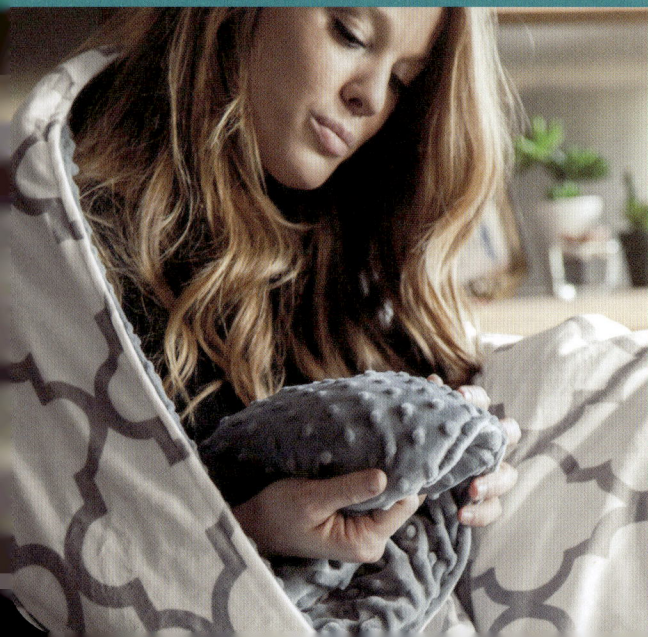

What We Know

Preliminary research suggests weighted blankets improve overall sleep quality through deep-pressure stimulation, a therapeutic technique thought to increase production of mood-boosting serotonin and reduce that of the stress hormone cortisol, according to the Sleep Foundation. It's generally safe to use if you're able to move it off yourself, but talk with your doctor first if you have sleep apnea or asthma. Most weighted blankets are between 10 and 30 pounds and experts generally recommend choosing one equal to 10% of your body weight. If you weigh 150 pounds, for example, opt for a 15-pound weighted blanket.

12 Monday

13 Tuesday

14 Wednesday

15 Thursday

16 Friday

17 Saturday

18 Sunday ●

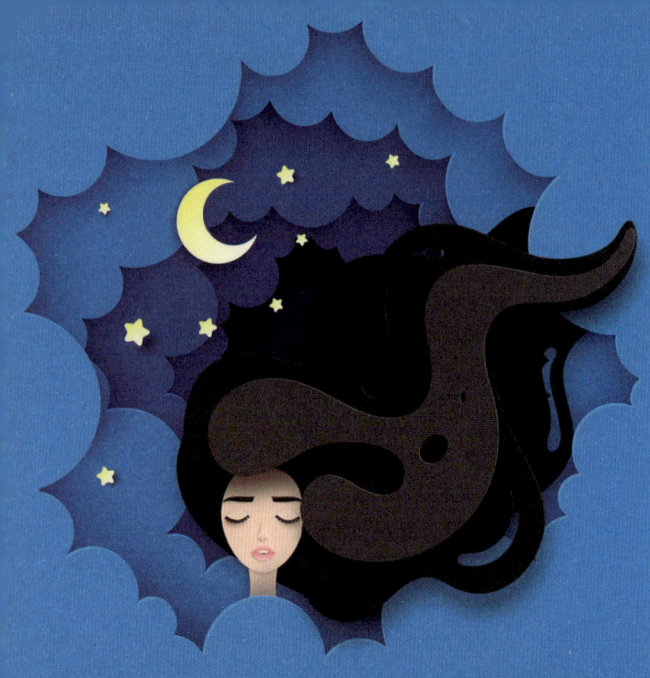

January 19–25

2026

M	T	W	T	F	S	S
			1	2	3	4
5	6	7	8	9	10	11
12	13	14	15	16	17	18
19	20	21	22	23	24	25
26	27	28	29	30	31	

MINIMIZE NIGHTMARES

If your otherwise peaceful sleep is interrupted regularly by vivid nightmares, it's helpful to know that two common culprits are stress and sleep deprivation, explains Alicia Roth, Ph.D., a clinical health psychologist specializing in behavioral sleep medicine at Cleveland Clinic. In addition to addressing those issues, consider a positive-imagery exercise before bed.

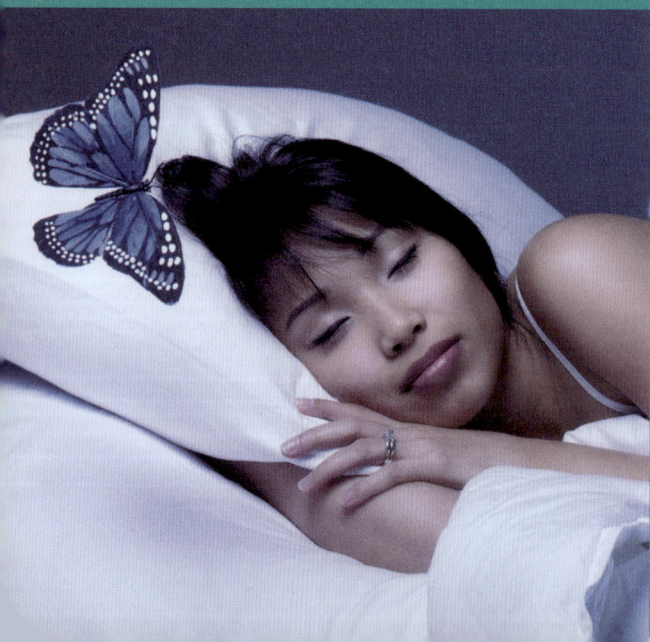

Try This Now

As you settle into bed for the night, walk yourself through an imaginary nature scene that brings you peace and comfort. Focus on what you would see, hear, and smell if you were really there and allow yourself time to imagine the fine details of the experience. "It's not always about getting rid of the bad stuff that appears in your nightmares; it's about adding in good, positive images for your brain to consume," says Roth. If your nightmares persist, see your doctor. You could have an underlying condition—anything from sleep apnea to PTSD—that could be manifesting as nightmares.

19 Monday Martin Luther King Jr. Day

20 Tuesday

21 Wednesday

22 Thursday

23 Friday

24 Saturday

25 Sunday

FEBRUARY 2026

MONDAY	TUESDAY	WEDNESDAY	THURSDAY
2 Groundhog Day	3	4	5
9 ◐	10	11	12 Lincoln's Birthday
16 Presidents' Day	17 Chinese New Year ●	18 Ramadan Begins	19
23	24 ◐	25	26

FRIDAY	SATURDAY	SUNDAY
		1 ○
6	7	8
13	14 Valentine's Day	15
20	21	22
27	28	

STRESS LESS

Get Some Sunlight. Even if it's frigid or snowy outside, exposing yourself to natural light will be worth the shivering—it helps keep your circadian rhythm on track for better sleep and a stronger immune system, aspects of good health that are especially important to attend to during cold and flu season.

JANUARY

M	T	W	T	F	S	S
			1	2	3	4
5	6	7	8	9	10	11
12	13	14	15	16	17	18
19	20	21	22	23	24	25
26	27	28	29	30	31	

MARCH

M	T	W	T	F	S	S
						1
2	3	4	5	6	7	8
9	10	11	12	13	14	15
16	17	18	19	20	21	22
23	24	25	26	27	28	29
30	31					

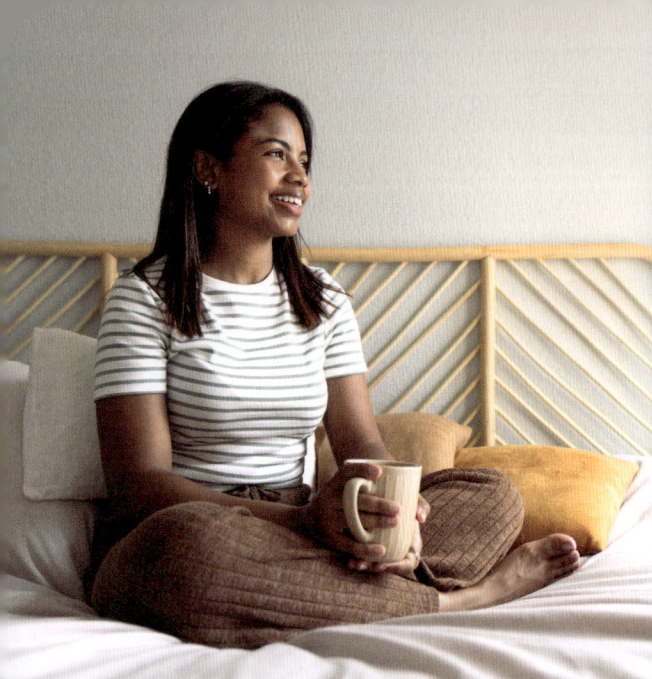

January 26–
February 1
2026

M	T	W	T	F	S	S
26	27	28	29	30	31	1
2	3	4	5	6	7	8
9	10	11	12	13	14	15
16	17	18	19	20	21	22
23	24	25	26	27	28	

TRY AN INPUT-FREE MORNING

Many of us spend breakfast catching up on the latest headlines. However, research has shown that especially as people get older, the onslaught of info can make it more difficult to process new information. Instead, try tuning out for the first hour of the day, giving your brain space to refresh itself so you can reset from all the noise and negativity of the previous day.

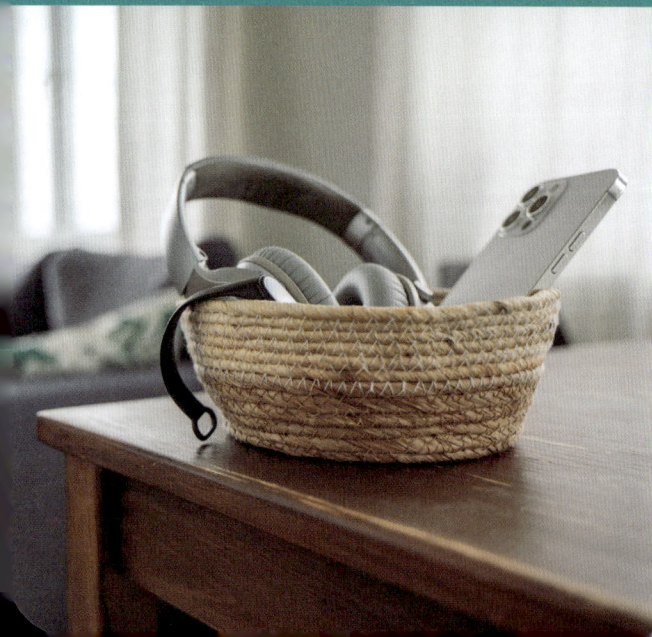

Why It Works

The problem with starting the day with the news cycle is that we tend to get caught up in information overload, says psychologist Amy Vigliotti, Ph.D., founder of SelfWorks in New York City. "You may start with researching one piece of information or checking in with one friend. Too often, though, you look up from your phone and find that hours have passed," she says. Not only is there too much info to process, but—these days especially—it tends to be bleak news. Most people take in about nine negative stories for every positive one, which essentially pumps up anxiety, keeping the brain in a state of high alert.

26 Monday ◐

27 Tuesday

28 Wednesday

29 Thursday

30 Friday

31 Saturday

1 Sunday ○

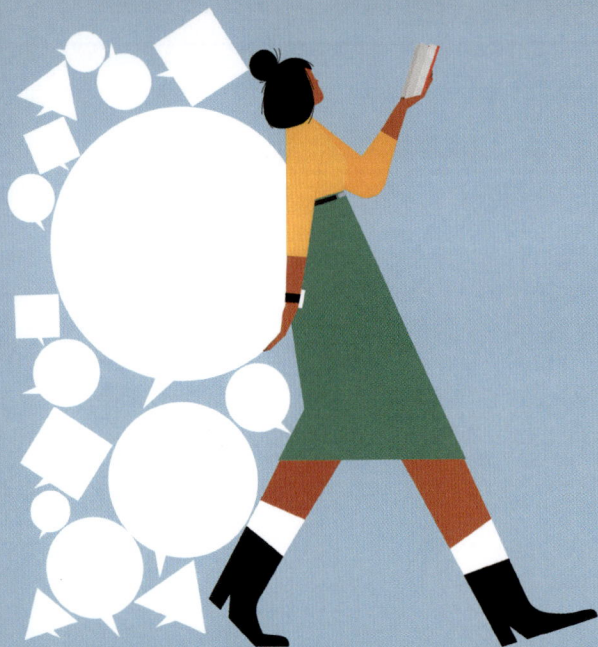

February
2–8
2026

M	T	W	T	F	S	S
						1
2	3	4	5	6	7	8
9	10	11	12	13	14	15
16	17	18	19	20	21	22
23	24	25	26	27	28	

TRY NOT TO MULTITASK

Yes, during a crazy busy day, it's hard to pay attention to just one thing at a time. But that is actually the golden ticket for memory. When you're multitasking, your attention is split between two (or three or four) things, and that's not ideal for focus. But when you concentrate on what you're doing, you're making it easier for your noggin to do its job.

What We Know

It's easy to feel busy as we talk on the phone while reading emails and packing up the kids' lunches. But switching tasks every few seconds is like pumping the gas and the brakes in your car, says Sandra Bond Chapman, Ph.D., chief director of the Center for BrainHealth at the University of Texas at Dallas and coleader of the BrainHealth Project. "When you multitask, you're breaking down your frontal networks and increasing the stress hormone cortisol, which makes your memory worse," she explains. Basically, if you try to do three things at once, you'll wind up doing none of them very well.

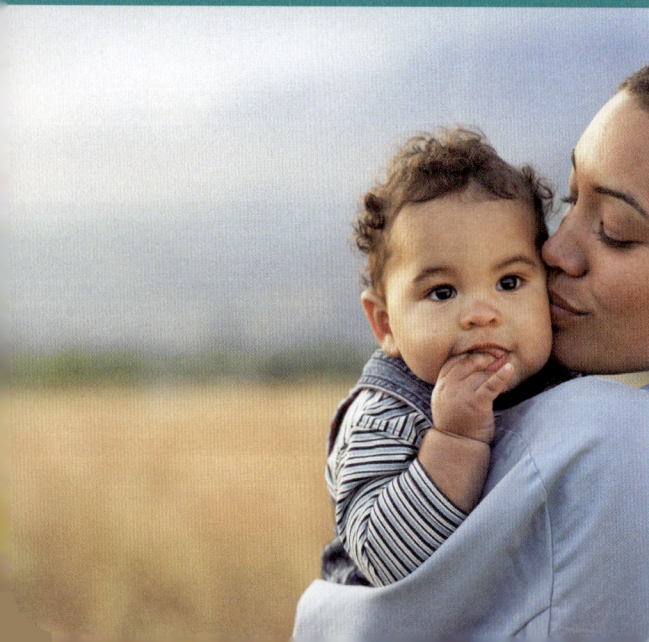

2 Monday Groundhog Day

3 Tuesday

4 Wednesday

5 Thursday

6 Friday

7 Saturday

8 Sunday

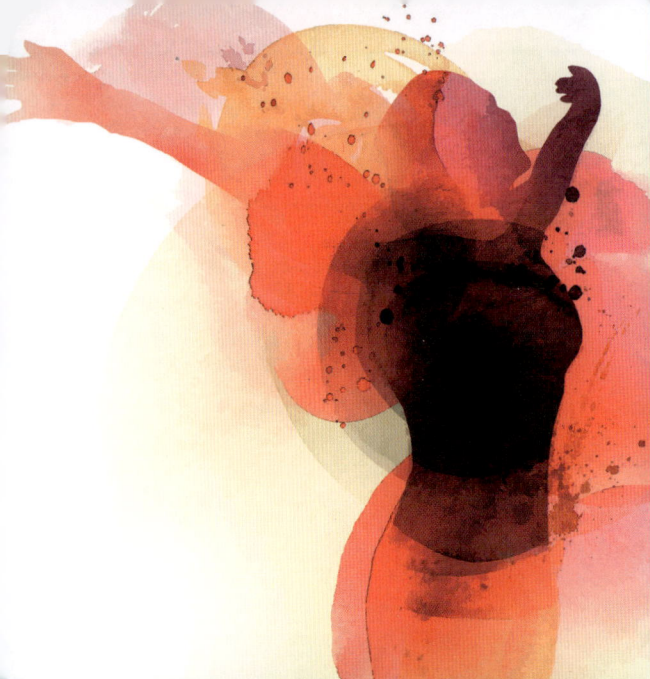

February
9–15
2026

M	T	W	T	F	S	S
						1
2	3	4	5	6	7	8
9	10	11	12	13	14	15
16	17	18	19	20	21	22
23	24	25	26	27	28	

MAKE SPACE FOR JOY

Consider getting rid of emotional baggage that's holding you back, such as that long-held grudge against your bestie-turned-frenemy. Grudges are the way your brain tricks you into feeling protected from future hurt, says Amy Vigliotti, Ph.D., founder of SelfWorks in New York City. However, it's hard to re-solve the feelings behind the grudge if you stay stuck in their rhythm.

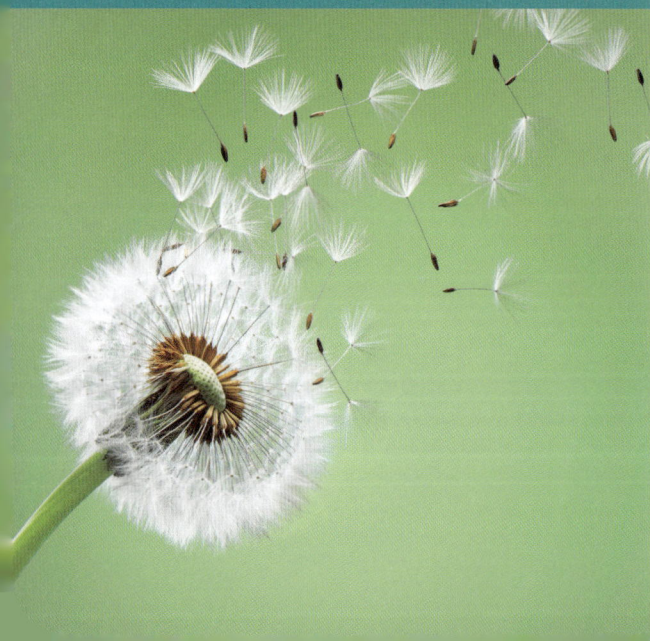

Try This Now

The real problem with this kind of chronic anger is that it may increase your risk of anxiety and depression. If your grudge is against a close friend or a relative, the answer may be as simple (though bravery-requiring) as asking for an apology or requesting more thoughtful behavior, says Vigliotti. Or you can try a visual cue to help your brain let go. Vigliotti recommends this exercise instead: Imagine yourself holding a white dandelion and telling it exactly what you're angry about, then blowing its seeds away. "There's something very freeing about that, because there's an actual physical action you experience as letting go," she says.

9 Monday ◑

10 Tuesday

11 Wednesday ○

12 Thursday Lincoln's Birthday

13 Friday

14 Saturday Valentine's Day

15 Sunday

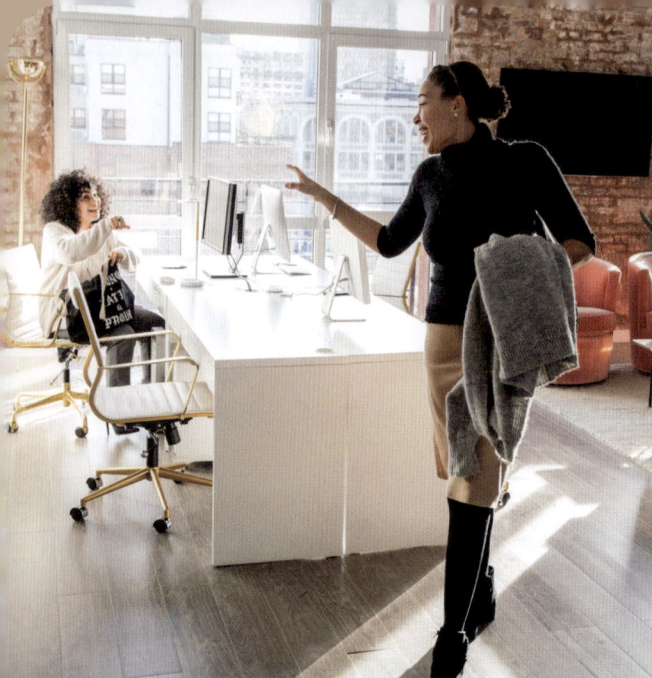

February
16–22

2026

M	T	W	T	F	S	S
						1
2	3	4	5	6	7	8
9	10	11	12	13	14	15
16	17	18	19	20	21	22
23	24	25	26	27	28	

MANAGE YOUR WORKLOAD

Most people ruminate about work at times, but when anxious thoughts are excessive and intrude into your personal life, it's time to address the issue. Research shows that when people detach themselves from work during their off hours, the result is increased energy levels, improved sleep, and better overall well-being.

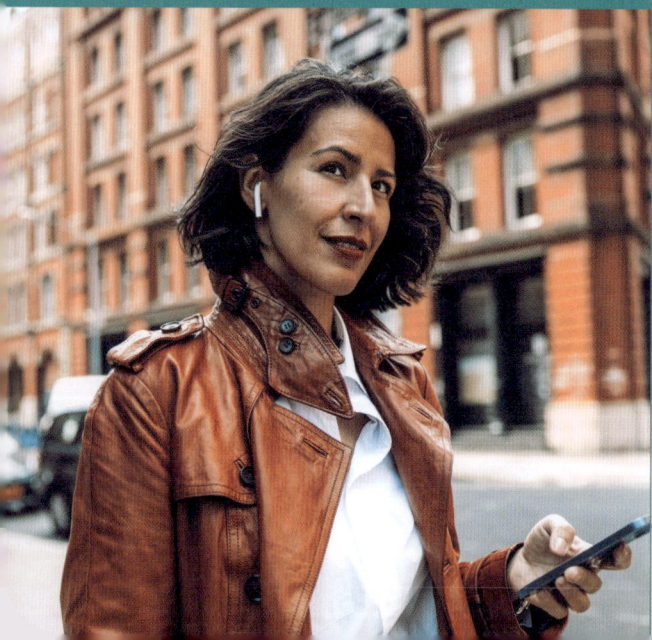

Here's What to Do

To dial back anxiety, train your mind to put a pin in the workweek. Start with brief stints of relaxation at the end of the workday, such as taking a short walk and noticing birds or listening to relaxing music during your homeward commute. Or try a separation ritual, such as consciously pushing in the desk chair and taking 10 deep breaths before letting go of the chair back. You can also try writing an accomplishments list at the end of each week before you start your Monday morning to-do list. One study revealed that people who ended the workweek on a positive note were better able to disconnect over the weekend than those who didn't.

16 Monday Presidents' Day

17 Tuesday ● Chinese New Year

18 Wednesday Ramadan Begins

19 Thursday

20 Friday

21 Saturday

22 Sunday

MARCH 2026

MONDAY	TUESDAY	WEDNESDAY	THURSDAY
2	3 Holi Begins ○	4	5
9	10	11 ◑	12
16	17 St. Patrick's Day	18	19 Eid al-Fitr Begins ●
23	24	25 ◐	26
30	31		

FRIDAY	SATURDAY	SUNDAY
		1
6	**7**	**8** Daylight Saving Time Begins
13	**14** Pi Day	**15** Laylat al-Qadr
20 First Day of Spring	**21**	**22**
27	**28**	**29** Palm Sunday

STRESS LESS

Plan a Getaway. Going on vacation is one of life's great pleasures—and science suggests it's good for our health. Studies show that taking time off has a positive effect on a person's mental state (more energy, less stress) and creativity, and simply having a vacay, staycation, or long weekend to look forward to contributes to overall well-being. What time-off excursions do you have coming up?

FEBRUARY

M	T	W	T	F	S	S
						1
2	3	4	5	6	7	8
9	10	11	12	13	14	15
16	17	18	19	20	21	22
23	24	25	26	27	28	

APRIL

M	T	W	T	F	S	S
		1	2	3	4	5
6	7	8	9	10	11	12
13	14	15	16	17	18	19
20	21	22	23	24	25	26
27	28	29	30			

February 23 – March 1

2026

M	T	W	T	F	S	S
23	24	25	26	27	28	1
2	3	4	5	6	7	8
9	10	11	12	13	14	15
16	17	18	19	20	21	22
23	24	25	26	27	28	29
30	31					

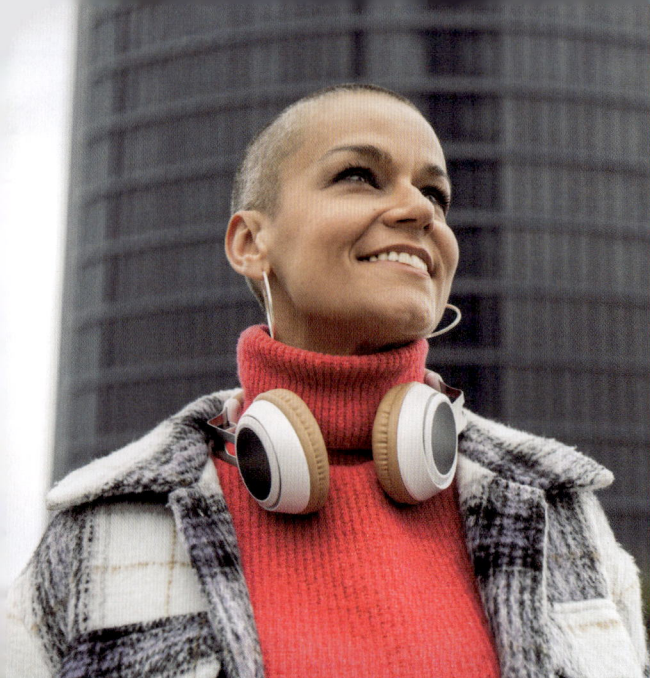

THIS WEEK I HOPE TO . . .

PRACTICE GRATITUDE

Being grateful is quite good for you. Research shows that appreciating blessings both big (say, a new baby in the family) and small (like hearing a favorite old song in your playlist) can boost happiness, and people who regularly practice gratitude tend to sleep better and have a lower risk of depression and anxiety.

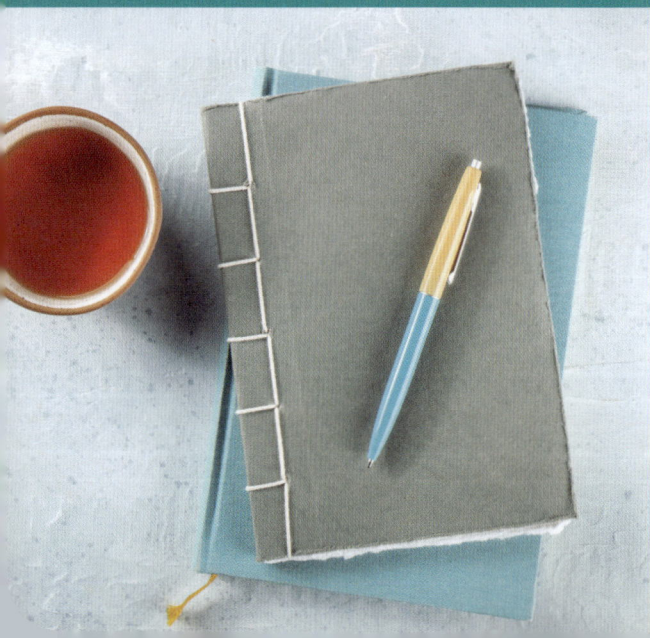

Try It Now

Writing down what you feel grateful for may help you dial back stress, studies suggest, because logging these moments prompts you to both remember and re-experience positive emotions. Beyond just writing down the things you're grateful for, it helps to vocalize them so you can hear yourself say them out loud. By the end of the week, return to your journal and read each day's entry aloud so your mind begins to override mental chatter you've inherited from other sources. There's never been a better time to start or nurture a gratitude ritual.

23 Monday

24 Tuesday

25 Wednesday

26 Thursday

27 Friday

28 Saturday

1 Sunday

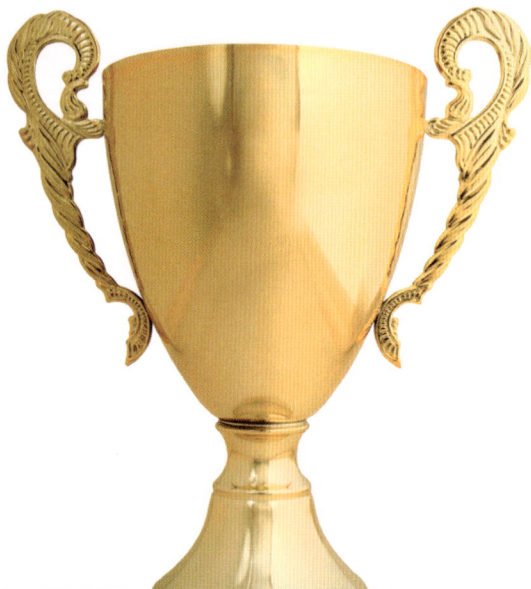

March
2–8
2026

M	T	W	T	F	S	S
						1
2	3	4	5	6	7	8
9	10	11	12	13	14	15
16	17	18	19	20	21	22
23	24	25	26	27	28	29
30	31					

I make the best lasagna

I have a real sense of style

I can think on my feet

I have beautiful eyes

Co-workers come to me with computer problems

I can do 20 push-ups (on my toes!)

Everyone says I'm funny

I am always there for my friends

I can finish the Sunday crossword

THINK ABOUT WHAT MAKES YOU SPECIAL

Social media can be a steady stream of humblebragging, but dwelling on where you fall short isn't helpful. "By learning to focus on ourselves instead of others, we can decrease our stress and anxiety and live a more purposeful and authentic life," says Renee Exelbert, Ph.D., a licensed psychologist and adjunct professor at New York University.

Here's What to Do

The same logic applies to material pursuits. "So much energy is spent chasing [physical] things we think will make us happy," says Amy Johnson, Ph.D., author of *The Little Book of Big Change*. "The next vacation, losing a few pounds—they never lead to lasting happiness." She says humans evolved to "recalibrate" quickly after events, so the happiness boost triggered by things outside of ourselves fades fast. Instead, try celebrating strengths and victories (even tiny ones!) without external validation. Teaching a niece how to read, having adventures with friends—intangibles like these give us real warm fuzzies.

2 Monday

3 Tuesday ○ Holi begins

4 Wednesday

5 Thursday

6 Friday

7 Saturday

8 Sunday Daylight Saving Time Begins

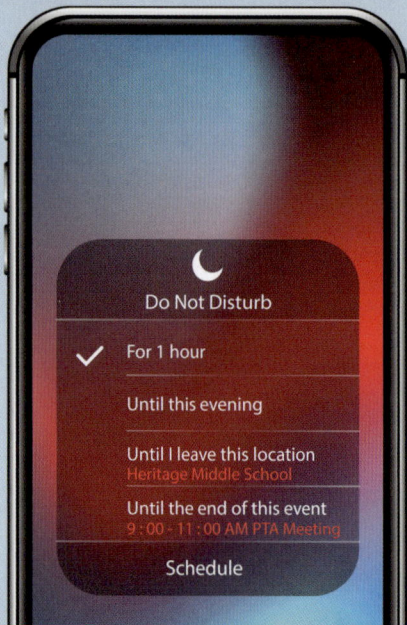

March
9–15
2026

M	T	W	T	F	S	S
						1
2	3	4	5	6	7	8
9	10	11	12	13	14	15
16	17	18	19	20	21	22
23	24	25	26	27	28	29
30	31					

TAKE A SCREEN BREAK

Your smartphone may be to blame for ramping up your anxiety: A recent San Francisco State University study found that the heaviest users of smartphones were also the most anxious, partly because the constant pings interrupted what they were doing and activated the same neural pathways in their brain that once alerted people to dangers such as lurking tigers.

What We Know

The relentless influx of news from traditional and social media doesn't help. "A few years ago, only the people who lived through a traumatic event were directly affected," says Catherine A. Sanderson, PhD., a professor of psychology at Amherst College and the author of *The Positive Shift.* "Now we can be part of the live experience and see things in a much more vivid way."

Learn to protect yourself: Shut off push notifications and take a break from social media. To keep worries from interfering with sleep, turn off screens an hour before bedtime and jot down your concerns so you can think about them tomorrow, not at 3 a.m.

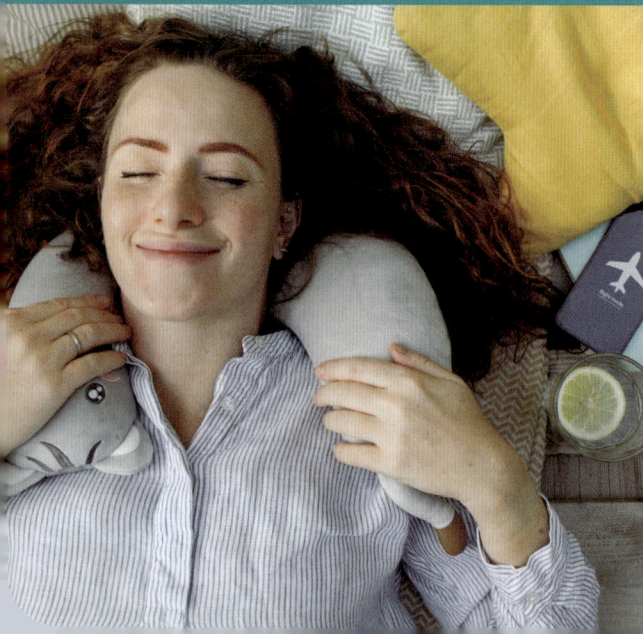

9 Monday

10 Tuesday

11 Wednesday ◑

12 Thursday

13 Friday

14 Saturday Pi Day

15 Sunday Laylat al-Qadr

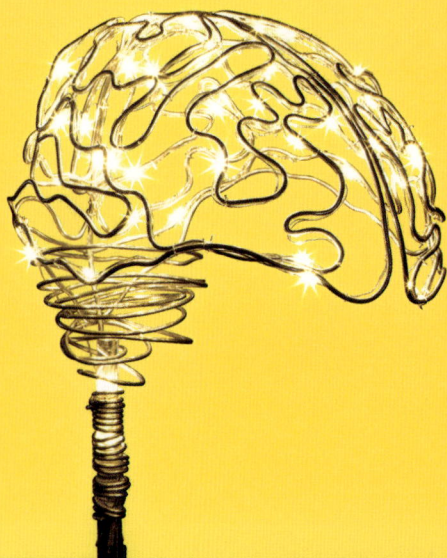

March 16–22

2026

M	T	W	T	F	S	S
						1
2	3	4	5	6	7	8
9	10	11	12	13	14	15
16	**17**	**18**	**19**	**20**	**21**	**22**
23	24	25	26	27	28	29
30	31					

GET A MASSAGE

Many of us have likely experienced a massage and other body services offered at a spa. These services are often the first go-to physical means to de-stress. It feels great while we are on the massage table and for hours afterward, yet we rarely speak about the impact on our biochemistry. Turns out there's quite a bit of science to explain why it feels so very good.

Why It Works

One review article looked at a number of medical studies that used massage therapy to address specific health conditions, including depression, pain syndromes, autoimmune diseases, job stress, and pregnancy. Unequivocally, the data revealed improvements in three hormones important in how we perceive stress.

Massage therapy decreased cortisol by 31% and activated two neurotransmitters: serotonin (our "happy" hormone) increased by 28% and dopamine (our "satisfaction" hormone) by 31%. It's important to make massage a regular part of your lifestyle because it is medically effective in alleviating stress.

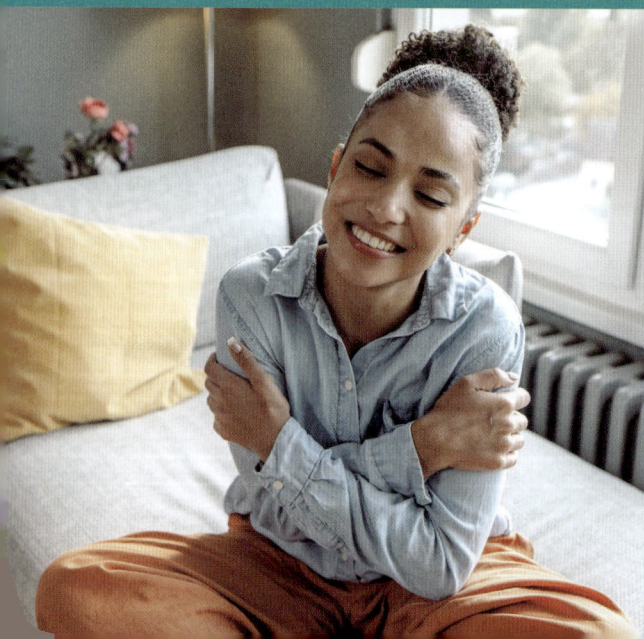

16 Monday

17 Tuesday St. Patrick's Day

18 Wednesday Eid al-Fitr Begins

19 Thursday ●

20 Friday First Day of Spring

21 Saturday

22 Sunday

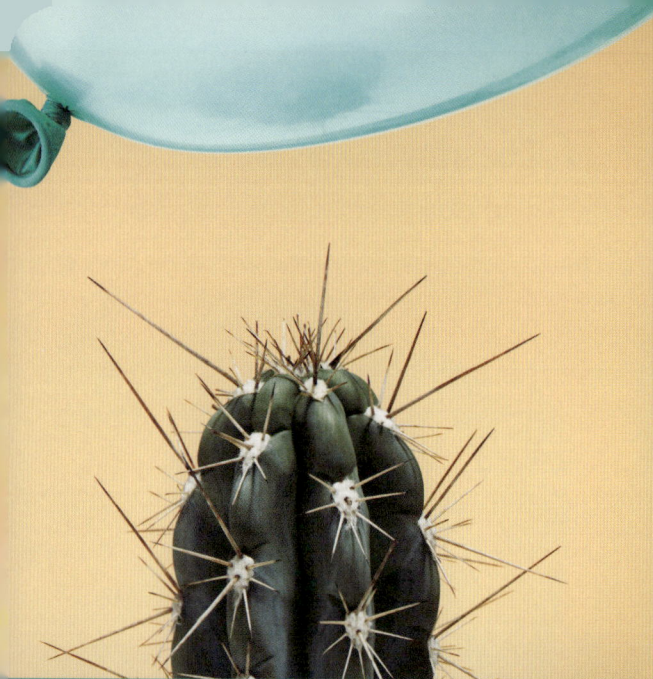

March
23–29
2026

M	T	W	T	F	S	S
						1
2	3	4	5	6	7	8
9	10	11	12	13	14	15
16	17	18	19	20	21	22
23	24	25	26	27	28	29
30	31					

CONFRONT YOUR ANXIETY

Though it's a natural reaction, avoidance may make your anxiety worse, says anxiety expert Haley Neidich, L.C.S.W. "Anxiety will insist on being felt," she says, and hiding from it can have secondary effects. In fact, a common treatment for anxiety is the opposite of avoidance: exposure therapy.

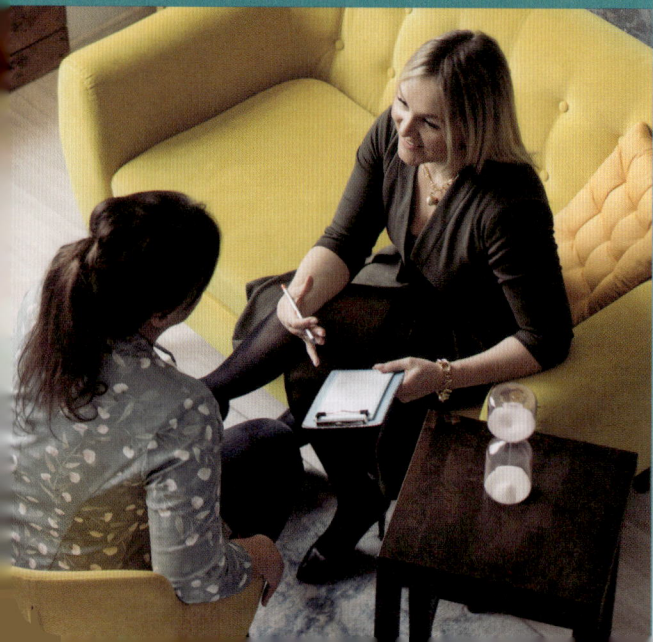

How It Works

Not speaking up in relationships, procrastinating, and avoiding social interactions or bills all have serious consequences, says Neidich. Exposure therapy works by helping people approach their fears in a safe environment—and, by doing so, learn that they can handle them. Sometimes the exposure is gradual, using virtual reality in the safety of a therapist's office or out in the real world. "Saying to yourself, 'Yup, I'm anxious; I feel it in my chest; I feel like I'm losing it' sounds simple, but it can reduce your symptoms immediately, and it puts you in a place of problem-solving rather than denying reality," Neidich says.

23 Monday

24 Tuesday

25 Wednesday ◑

26 Thursday

27 Friday

28 Saturday

29 Sunday Palm Sunday

SPRING
FOCUS ON
FITNESS

Just about any physical activity you choose is guaranteed to be a proven stress reliever and mood booster, so take time this season to reset your fitness goals. Stretching, in particular, is a great way to start. Not only will a head-to-toe stretch do wonders for your muscles, but there are also significant ways stretching can lower your stress levels. Plus, the deep belly breaths, which you'll take while performing the Pilates moves provided in this section, can have a calming effect.

The best part is that these moves require virtually no equipment, just an exercise mat and a sturdy wall says Kathryn Ross-Nash, a pilates instructor and author of *Prevention's Stretch Away Pain.* That means in just a few minutes you can stretch your way to a better physical and mental place whether you're at home, in an office, or on the go. Let's get started!

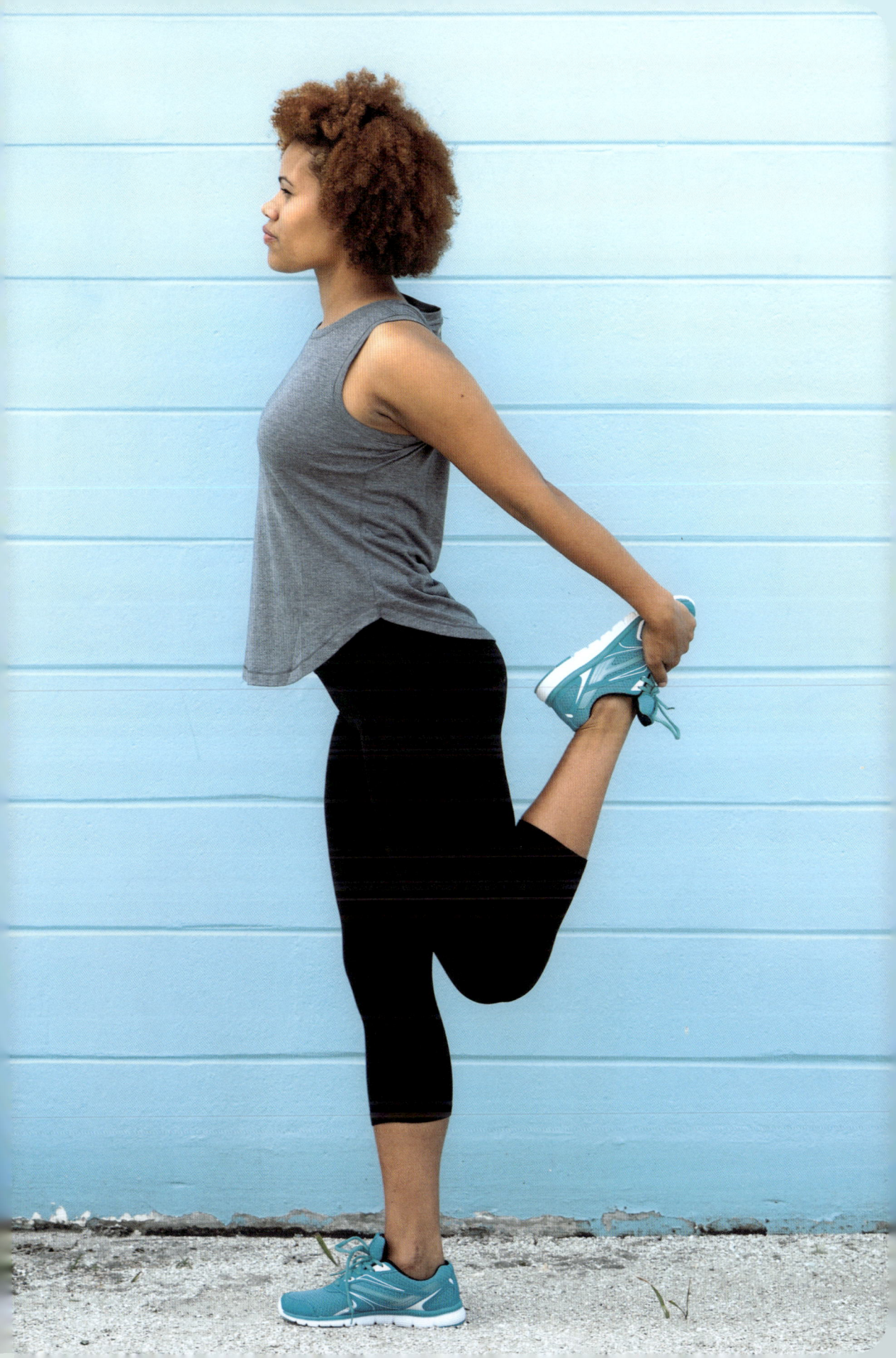

Stretch Away Stress

Pilates is perhaps best known for strengthening and toning, but many of the exercises will also give you a good stretch. You'll bend and twist and reach for your toes while sculpting lean muscle. In fact, research has shown that people who do Pilates just three times a week have increased hamstring flexibility, which is especially important to avoid injury from walking or running. Better flexibility can reduce your risk of injury in general by relieving stiff muscles, thereby allowing you to move with more control. Take 10 minutes to breathe deeply and create space in your body with these Pilates moves.

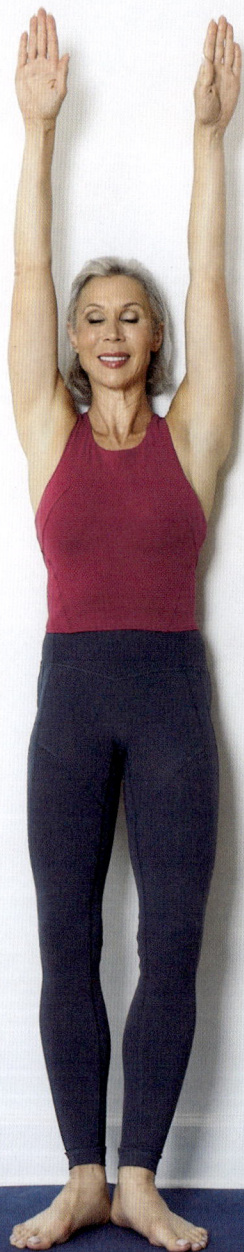

Rolldown Arm Circle

SETUP Stand with your back leaning against the wall, heels together and about six inches from the wall. Your feet should be one hand-width apart. Soften your knees, lengthen your spine, and place your arms by your sides.

1 Inhale deeply and lift your arms overhead, palms facing forward.

2 Exhale, squeezing all the air out of your lungs as you lower your arms and fold forward from the waist, tucking your chin into your chest.

3 Inhale, lift your arms forward, and roll your torso up the wall from your waist. Bring your arms overhead as the back of your head returns to touch the wall.

4 Repeat, reversing the movement so you start bent over and lift your arms as you roll up.

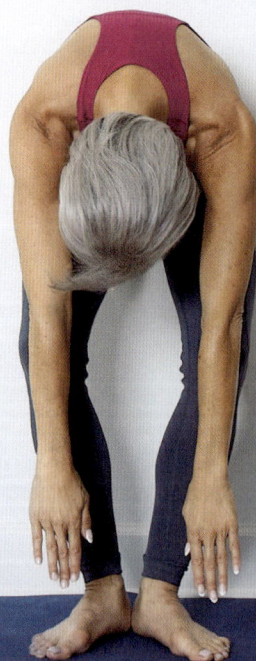

Cat and Cow with Straight Knees

SETUP Stand with your hands against the wall at shoulder height. Walk your feet back until your torso is flat like a tabletop. Keep your legs hip-width apart.

1 Inhale and press your hands to the wall, legs straight but not locked.

2 Roll your shoulders to your ears and circle them back and down to lift your head. As your head lifts, exhale and arch your entire spine, lifting your chest forward.

3 Inhale and return to tabletop position.

4 Exhale and round forward, arching your spine like a scared cat, tucking your chin to your chest.

5 Inhale and return to tabletop position.

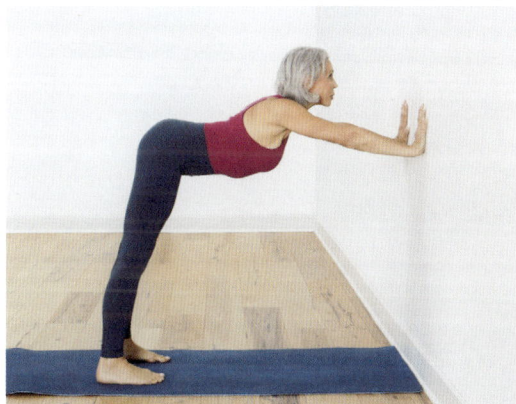

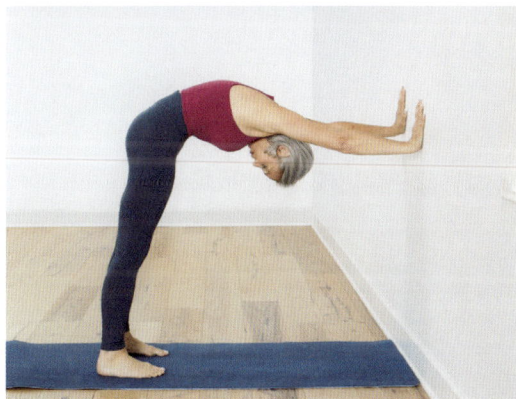

Side Bend

SETUP Stand with your left side to the wall, arms at your sides and feet slightly past hip-width apart.

1 Lift your right arm up and bend to the left to reach to the wall; while reaching, bring your left palm to the wall.

2 Reverse the action and lift your palm off the wall as you return to an upright position.

3 Repeat on the other side.

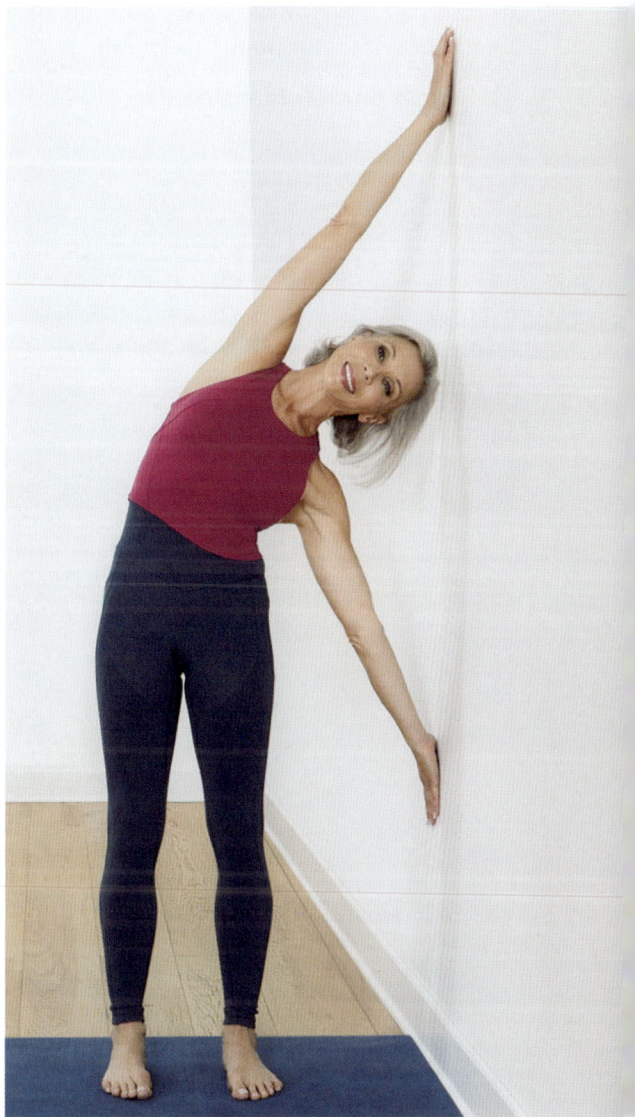

Spine Twist

SETUP Sit with the right side of your body next to a wall, your left knee bent up and your right leg straight.

1 Reach your arms forward with palms touching, keeping them at shoulder height. Your right shoulder should be touching the wall.

2 Inhale and open your left arm to the side while turning your head to the left. Exhale and twist your torso to the left. Reach your hands away from each other to increase the stretch. Inhale and return to center with your palms touching.

3 Repeat on the other side.

Single-Leg Stretch

SETUP Lie on a mat and place your feet flat on the wall, hip-width apart, knees bent 90 degrees. Place your arms down by your sides. Keep your back long and flat on the mat.

1 Inhale fully, then exhale and tip your tailbone up to lift your pelvis off the mat.

2 Inhale fully, then exhale while bringing your right knee in to your chest. Hold your right shin with your hands and press your leg toward your chest for three seconds.

3 Inhale and return your right foot to the wall. Lower your tailbone down to the mat.

4 Repeat with your left leg.

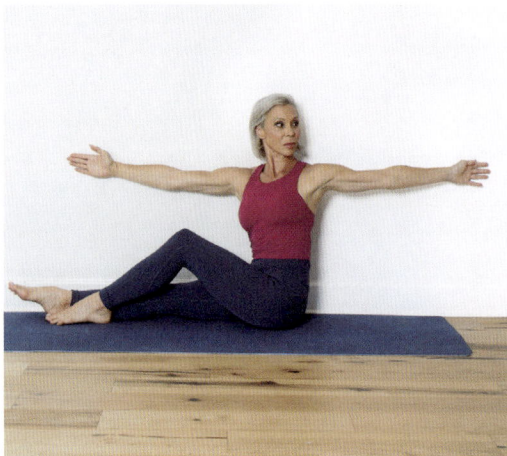

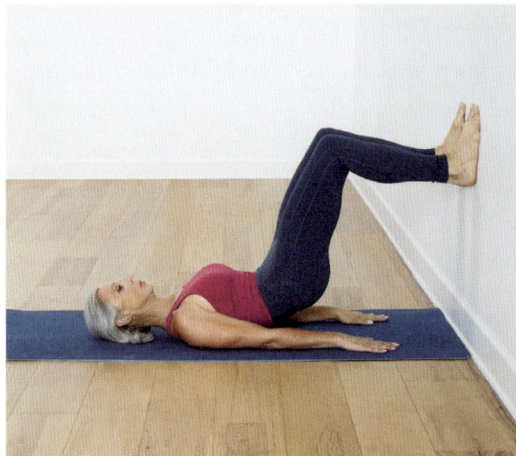

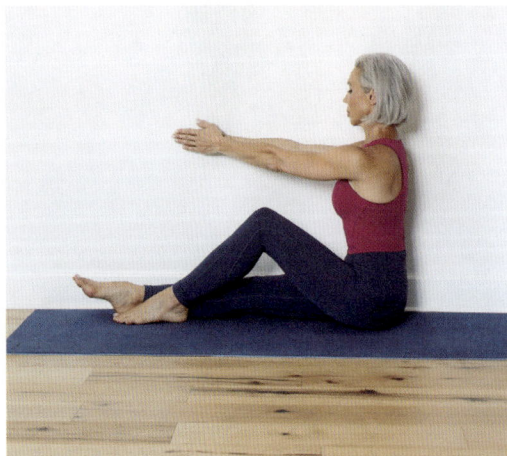

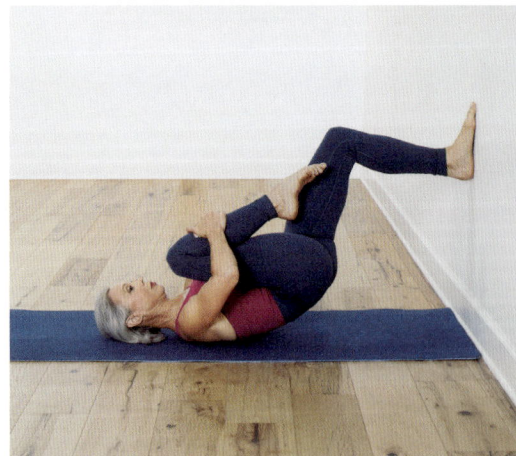

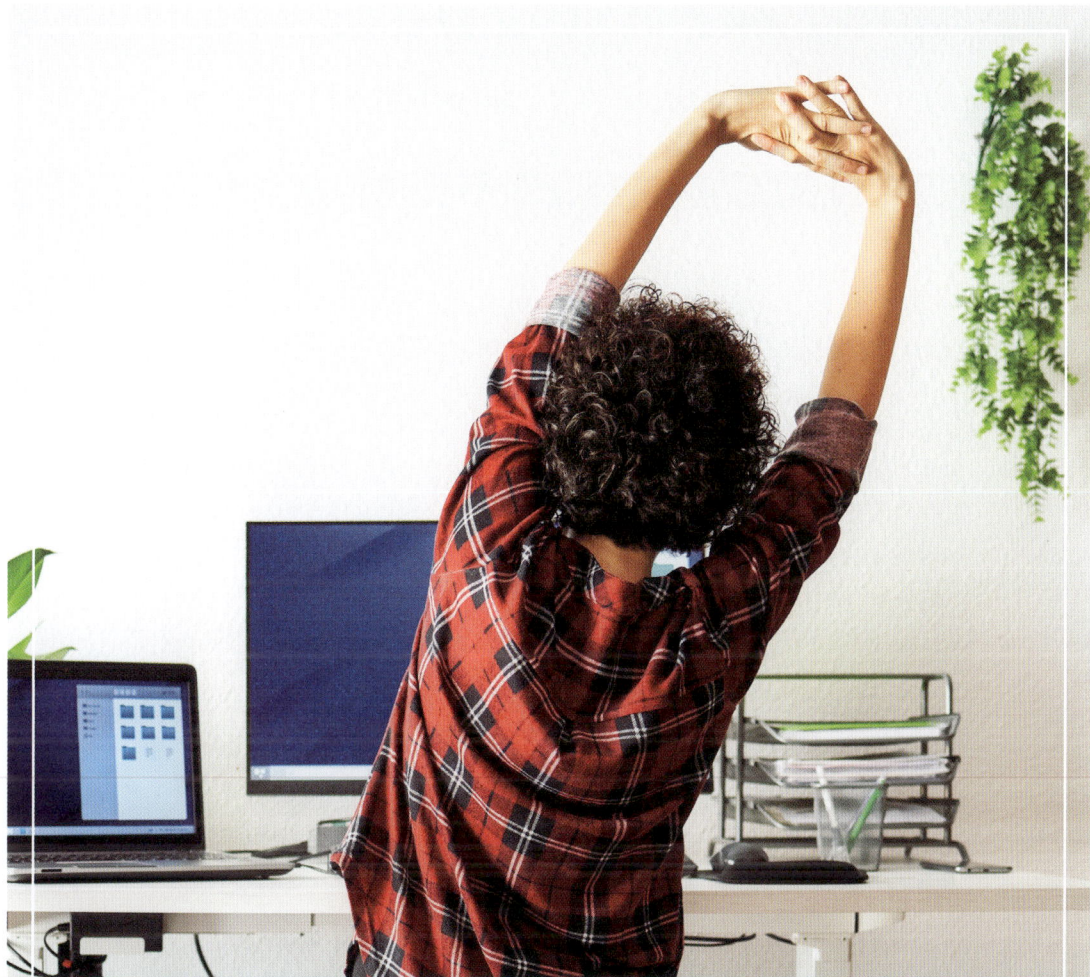

Should You Stretch at a Certain Time of Day?

Stretching is a helpful activity no matter when you fit it into your schedule, though your range of motion will be better if you warm up your muscles first with exercise, a short walk, or a warm bath or shower. But it's beneficial at any time of day.

"Stretching first thing in the morning can help promote better posture, mobility, and movement throughout the day," says Rachel Tavel, P.T., D.P.T., C.S.C.S., author of *Stretch Yourself Healthy: Easy Routines to Relieve Pain, Boost Energy, and Feel Refreshed.* "Midday stretching is a great way to get out of a postural slump. And stretching in the evening can help you wind down, tune into where tension has developed, and breathe away stress." It's also fine to squeeze stretching in here and there throughout the day when while you're waiting for your toast, watching TV, or showering. Every bit counts!

APRIL 2026

MONDAY	TUESDAY	WEDNESDAY	THURSDAY
		1 April Fools' Day Passover Begins	2 ○
6	7	8	9
13	14	15 Tax Day	16
20	21	22 Earth Day	23
27	28	29	30

FRIDAY	SATURDAY	SUNDAY
3 Good Friday	**4**	**5** Easter Sunday
10 ◑	**11**	**12**
17 ●	**18**	**19**
24 Arbor Day ◐	**25**	**26**

MOVE WELL

Tap into Optimism.
Are you a glass-half-full or a glass-half-empty person? People who have a hopeful viewpoint are healthier mentally and physically and live longer, happier lives, research suggests. Negative thinking is not entirely in your DNA: You can shift your perspective, and mindfully focusing on things like a fresh cup of coffee or a sunny afternoon can help make that glass feel a little more full.

MARCH

M	T	W	T	F	S	S
						1
2	3	4	5	6	7	8
9	10	11	12	13	14	15
16	17	18	19	20	21	22
23	24	25	26	27	28	29
30	31					

MAY

M	T	W	T	F	S	S
				1	2	3
4	5	6	7	8	9	10
11	12	13	14	15	16	17
18	19	20	21	22	23	24
25	26	27	28	29	30	31

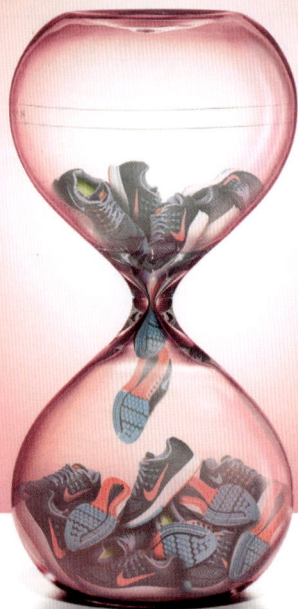

March 30–April 5

2026

M	T	W	T	F	S	S
30	**31**	**1**	**2**	**3**	**4**	**5**
6	7	8	9	10	11	12
13	14	15	16	17	18	19
20	21	22	23	24	25	26
27	28	29	30			

MAKE A MOVEMENT PLAN

How much movement do you get over the average day or week? If you're not regularly getting at least 150 minutes of moderate exercise or 75 minutes of vigorous exercise per week, as recommended by the CDC, come up with a concrete plan for how you'll reach that goal or work toward it over time.

Here's What to Do

Consider scheduling exercise sessions like appointments on your calendar or having a workout buddy who'll hold you accountable. Regular exercise becomes a habit if you make it a priority, says Wendy Bazilian, Dr.P.H., R.D.N., author of *The Super-FoodsRx Diet*.

Also, you'll be more likely to stick with your exercise goals when you do an activity you love. If jogging or using the weight machines at the gym doesn't sound fun to you, find something that does. Consistency is key for reaping the biggest benefits from exercise.

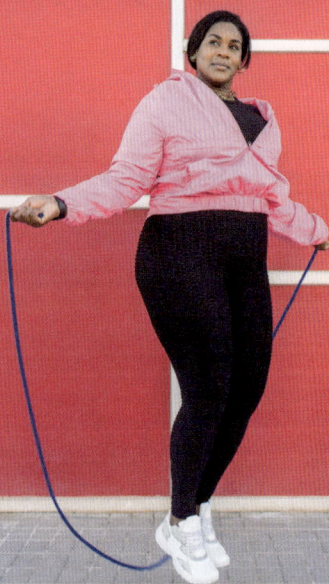

30 Monday

31 Tuesday

1 Wednesday April Fools' Day
Passover Begins

2 Thursday ○

3 Friday Good Friday

4 Saturday

5 Sunday Easter Sunday

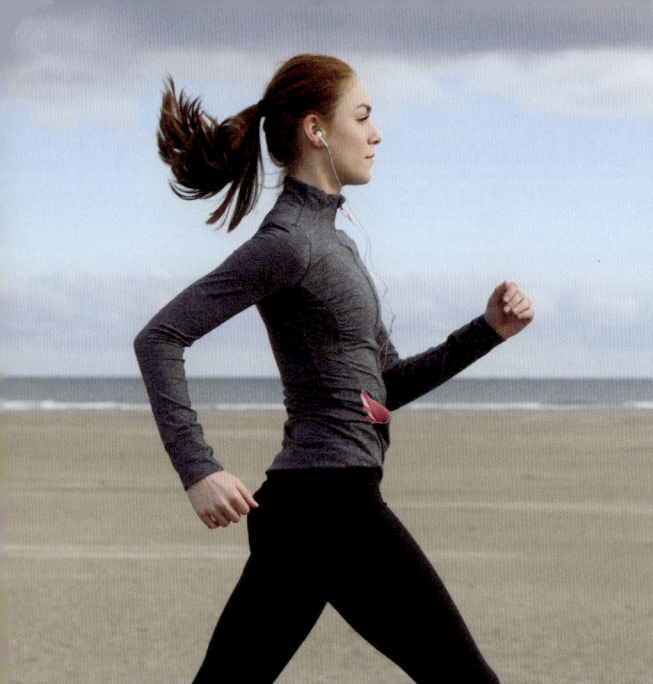

April
6–12
2026

M	T	W	T	F	S	S
		1	2	3	4	5
6	7	8	9	10	11	12
13	14	15	16	17	18	19
20	21	22	23	24	25	26
27	28	29	30			

TRY POWER WALKING

Walking is a foolproof stress buster. But it can be so much more than just putting one foot in front of the other. Power walking is all about getting your heart rate up. The hasty pace causes your brain to release chemicals called endorphins that stimulate relaxation and improve mood. Plus, you'll get relaxation benefits from all the deep breathing.

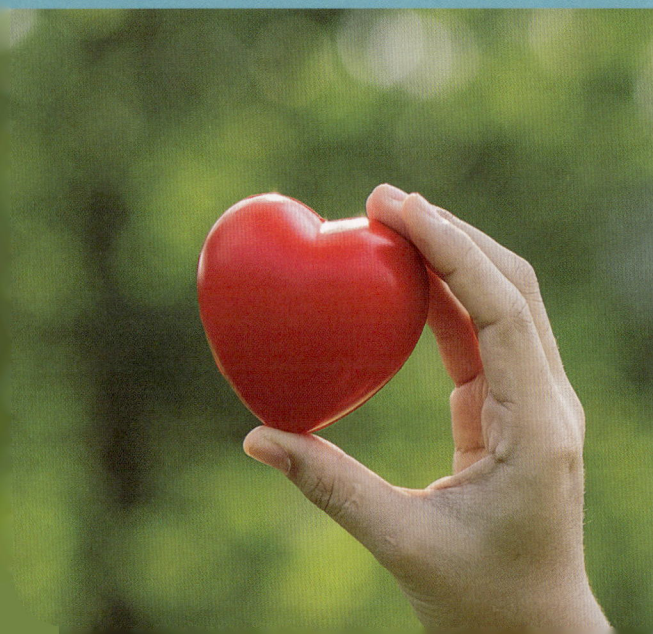

Try It Now

Start at a pace somewhere between a really quick walk and a very slow run. Keep your back straight and avoid hunching forward. While walking, move your arms in rhythm with the movement of your feet, back and forth, just like you would during a regular walk but faster. Your stride may feel awkward at first, but once you begin to work this into your routine, you will get the hang of it.

Remember, too, to set achievable goals. Start small (even just once a week for 20 minutes is a great start!), then eventually aim to walk three days a week for 20 minutes or longer, ideally outdoors.

6 Monday

7 Tuesday

8 Wednesday

9 Thursday

10 Friday ◑

11 Saturday

12 Sunday

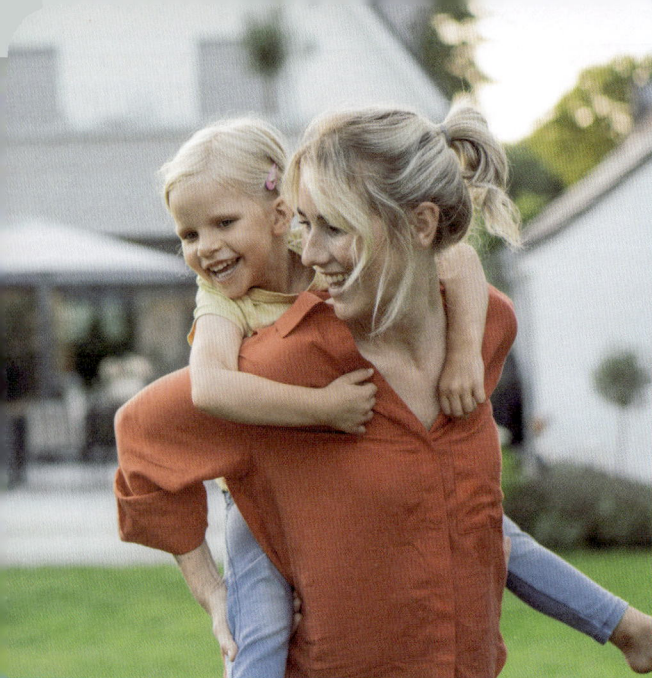

April
13–19
2026

M	T	W	T	F	S	S
		1	2	3	4	5
6	7	8	9	10	11	12
13	14	15	16	17	18	19
20	21	22	23	24	25	26
27	28	29	30			

STRETCH AWAY BACK PAIN

Stretching is a powerful painkiller. All your muscles, bones, and tendons are connected, so pain in one body part can affect another. With stretching, you can loosen multiple areas at once. Try this back-centric move from *Prevention*'s *Stretch Away Pain* by Kathryn Ross-Nash.

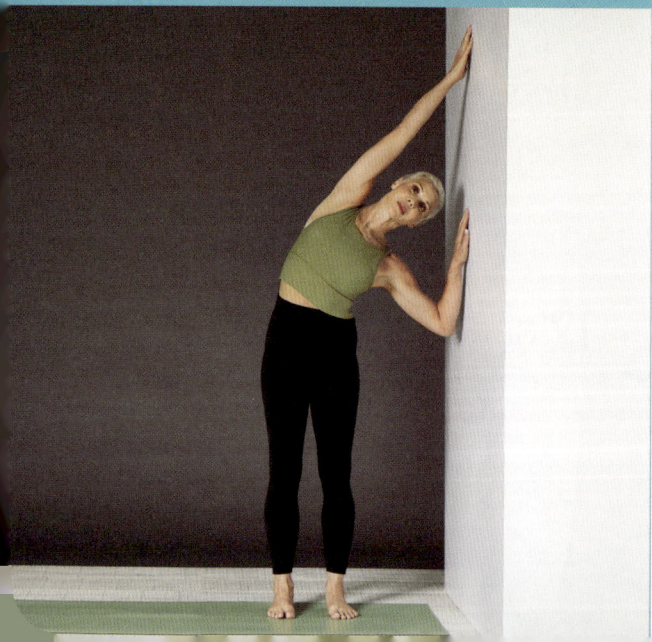

Here's What to Do

1. Stand sideways about one foot from a wall, legs sit-bone-width apart and toes forward. Place your left hand on a wall at shoulder height (elbow bent and down), slightly in front of your shoulder. Bend your right arm to bring your thumb in front of your right armpit, palm facing the wall.

2. Extend your right arm straight up, pulling your stomach in, and reach your right arm toward the wall, stretching the right side of your body. Hold for three counts.

3. Return to starting position. Repeat two times, then reset and repeat on the opposite side.

13 Monday

14 Tuesday

15 Wednesday Tax Day

16 Thursday

17 Friday ●

18 Saturday

19 Sunday

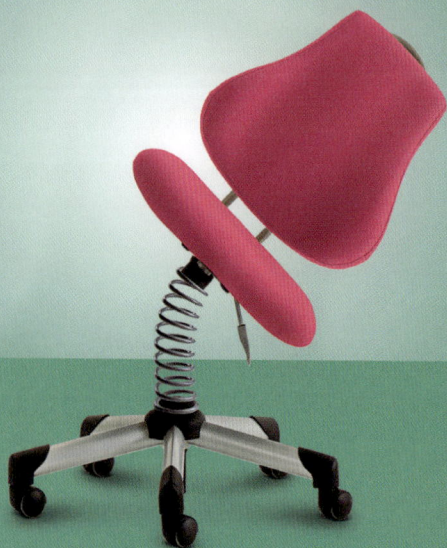

April
20–26
2026

M	T	W	T	F	S	S
		1	2	3	4	5
6	7	8	9	10	11	12
13	14	15	16	17	18	19
20	21	22	23	24	25	26
27	28	29	30			

SPEND LESS TIME SITTING

Science keeps trying to warn us: Sitting is terrible for you. Sedentary behavior is associated with an increased chance for chronic diseases such as heart disease, type 2 diabetes, and cancer as well as a potentially shorter life span. The good news is that research also suggests that finding reasons to move throughout your day could be an antidote.

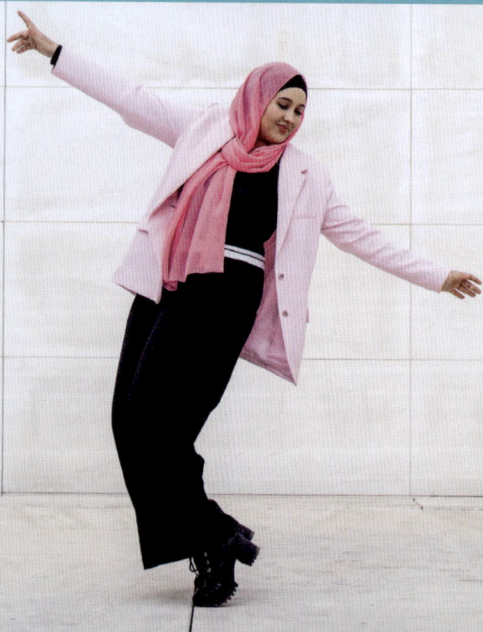

Try It Now

It's easy to miss regular alarms, so surprise yourself into standing. Set an hourly alarm for random times like 12:41 and 1:43. When you get an alert, have a five-minute "movement snack," says Lindsey Benoit O'Connell, founder of The LAB Wellness. You could:

- Have a one-song dance party
- Stretch
- Refill your water bottle
- Take a detour to the bathroom
- Do jumping jacks, squats, or pushups

20 Monday

21 Tuesday

22 Wednesday Earth Day

23 Thursday

24 Friday ◗ Arbor Day

25 Saturday

26 Sunday

MAY 2026

MONDAY	TUESDAY	WEDNESDAY	THURSDAY
4	5 Cinco de Mayo	6	7
11	12	13	14
18	19	20	21
25 Memorial Day	26	27	28

FRIDAY	SATURDAY	SUNDAY
1 May Day ○	**2**	**3**
8	**9** ◑	**10** Mother's Day
15	**16** Armed Forces Day ●	**17**
22	**23** ◑	**24**
29	**30**	**31** ○

MOVE WELL

Do something that's just for you. Regular "me time" can help with stress relief, but we don't always make it a priority. This is Mental Health Awareness Month, so there's no better time to hit reset and commit to doing a little self-care each day.

APRIL

M	T	W	T	F	S	S
	1	2	3	4	5	
6	7	8	9	10	11	12
13	14	15	16	17	18	19
20	21	22	23	24	25	26
27	28	29	30			

JUNE

M	T	W	T	F	S	S
1	2	3	4	5	6	7
8	9	10	11	12	13	14
15	16	17	18	19	20	21
22	23	24	25	26	27	28
29	30					

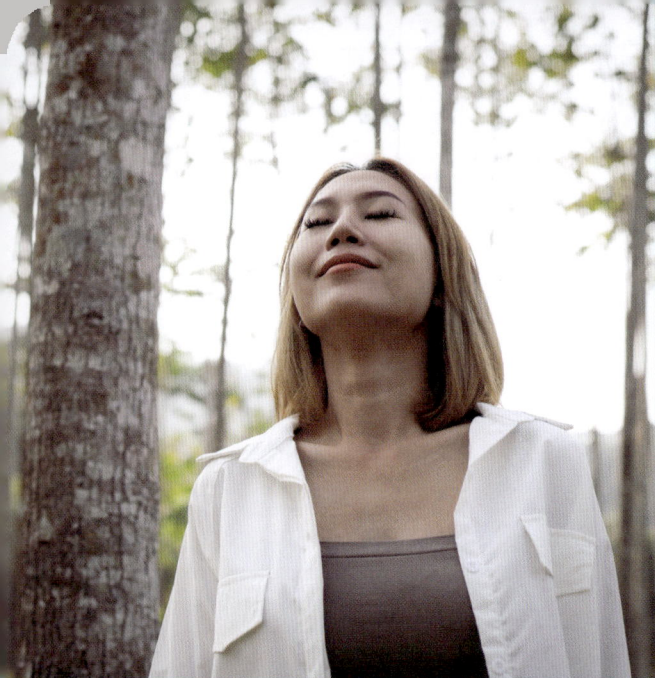

April 27– May 3

2026

M	T	W	T	F	S	S
27	28	29	30	1	2	3
4	5	6	7	8	9	10
11	12	13	14	15	16	17
18	19	20	21	22	23	24
25	26	27	28	29	30	31

GET OUTSIDE!

It's easy to spend the entire day indoors—working in an office, doing chores around the house, and shuttling between the two inside a car or bus. Today, even if you live in a concrete jungle, schedule a half-hour walk outdoors, preferably in a place where you can see at least a hint of nature's wonders.

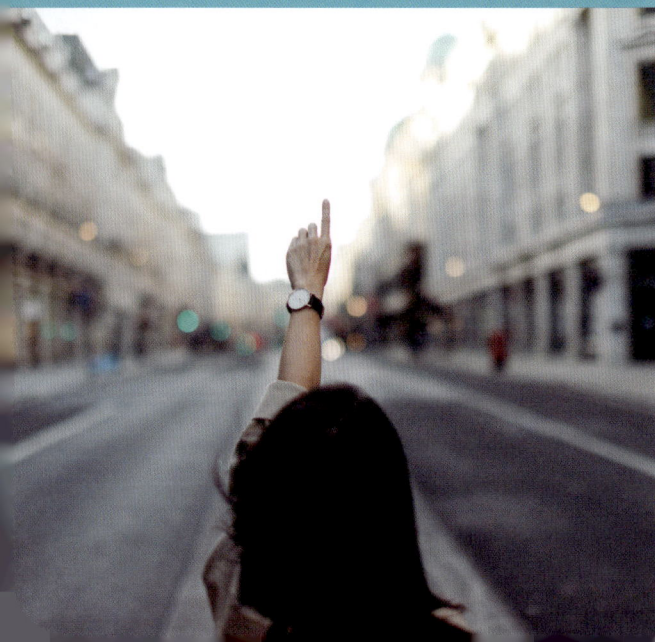

What We Know

"Walking can help you calm your senses and reengage or reset after a stressful morning or a stressful day," says Judy Ho, Ph.D., a board-certified neuropsychologist and the author of *Stop Self-Sabotage*.

For an added boost, try this breathing exercise while you walk. Imagine a box in front of your face and use your finger to trace the border: Breathe in as your finger goes up one side, hold your breath as it goes across the top, exhale as your finger moves down the other side, and hold again as it continues across the bottom to close out the rectangle. Repeat that five to 10 times.

27 Monday

28 Tuesday

29 Wednesday

30 Thursday

1 Friday ○ May Day

2 Saturday

3 Sunday

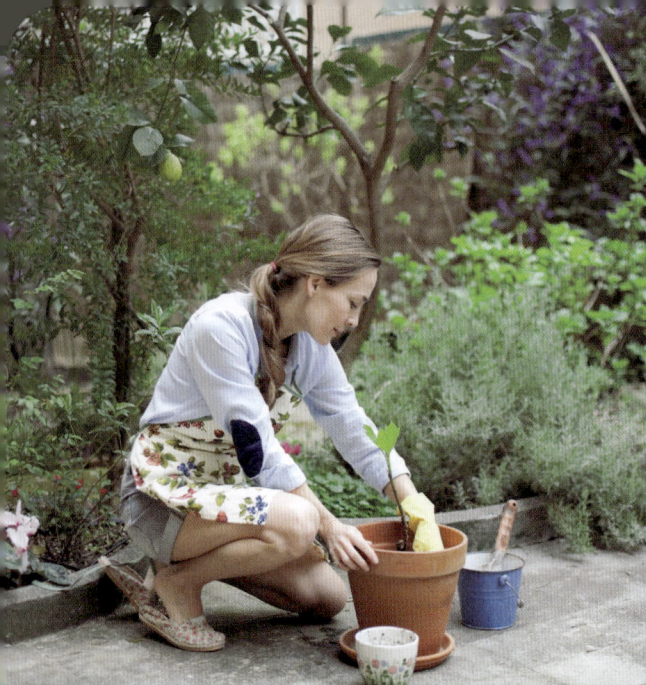

May
4–10
2026

M	T	W	T	F	S	S
				1	2	3
4	5	6	7	8	9	10
11	12	13	14	15	16	17
18	19	20	21	22	23	24
25	26	27	28	29	30	31

START A GARDEN

Here's some good news for gardeners: Getting down and dirty can spruce up your yard *and* your health! Research has dug up mental health benefits, showing that gardening may help ease stress, depression, and anxiety while enhancing happiness and well-being. Whether you're realizing your dream landscape or just starting out, here's how to boost your mood.

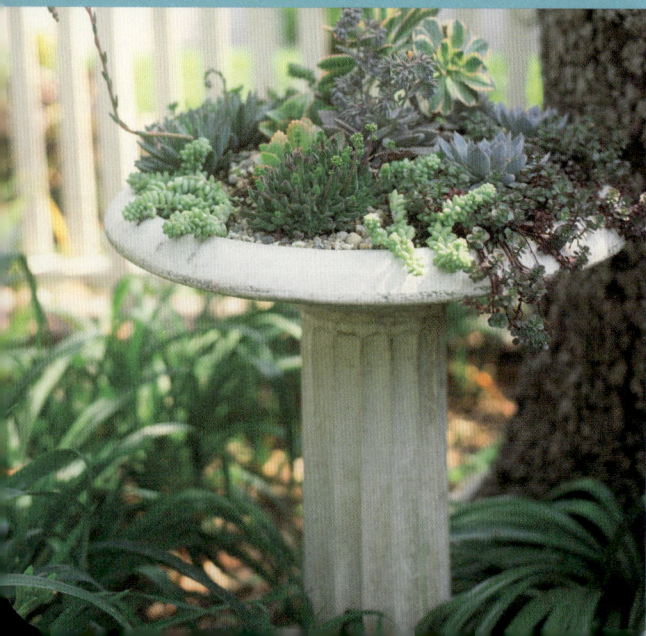

Here's What to Do

When making a plan, remember to think beyond the plants—add stones, a birdbath, or other garden decor that brings you joy. And don't stress about planting everything in one day. As with traditional exercise, overdoing it may leave you sore or strained (don't forget to take breaks to stretch and hydrate).

If you don't have a patch of ground to call your own, see if you can volunteer at or rent a plot in a community garden, and explore other related activities such as volunteer initiatives to beautify a park. All are great ways to reap the benefits of both gardening and socializing!

4 Monday

5 Tuesday Cinco de Mayo

6 Wednesday

7 Thursday

8 Friday

9 Saturday ◑

10 Sunday Mother's Day

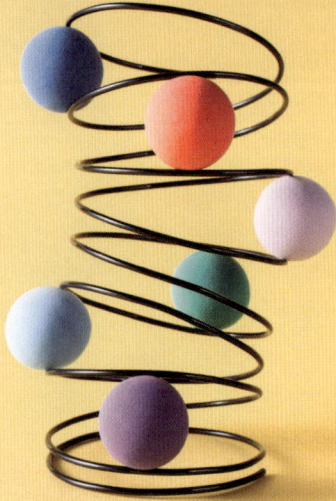

May
11–17
2026

M	T	W	T	F	S	S
				1	2	3
4	5	6	7	8	9	10
11	12	13	14	15	16	17
18	19	20	21	22	23	24
25	26	27	28	29	30	31

STAVE OFF BACK PAIN

Stress absolutely can cause back pain. In one large study, severe stress was associated with a nearly threefold increase in risk for chronic low-back pain. That's because the stress response causes muscles to tense up, which can affect your head, neck, shoulders, and spine.

What We Know

Stress can also negatively impact sleep, make posture worse, and cause inflammation throughout the body, says Jonathan Guymon, D.C., a chiropractor with Gateway to Wellness Chiropractic in Cedar Park, TX. "Low-back pain issues are often issues of a sedentary, high-stress lifestyle," he says. So get up and move, especially your spine.

Seek treatment if you have severe pain that doesn't decrease after three days and/or travels down your leg, changes in bowel or bladder function, or numbness, tingling, or weakness. Those can be symptoms of a herniated disc or another condition that may not get better on its own.

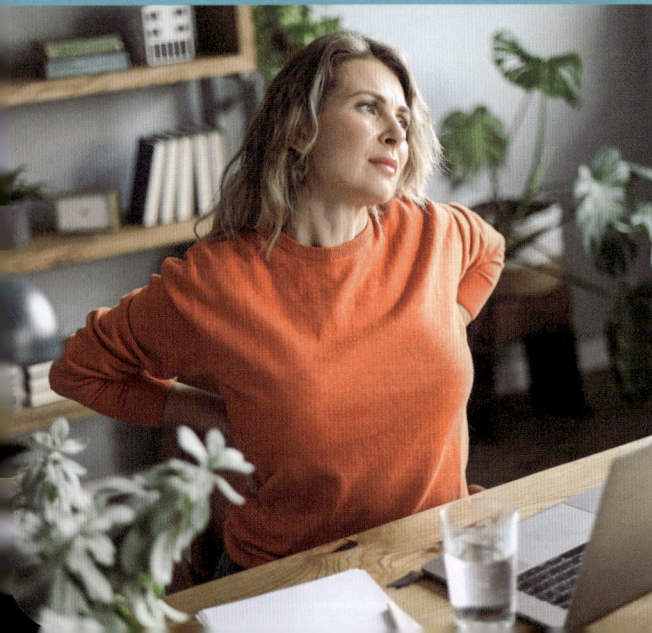

11 Monday

12 Tuesday

13 Wednesday

14 Thursday

15 Friday

16 Saturday ● Armed Forces Day

17 Sunday

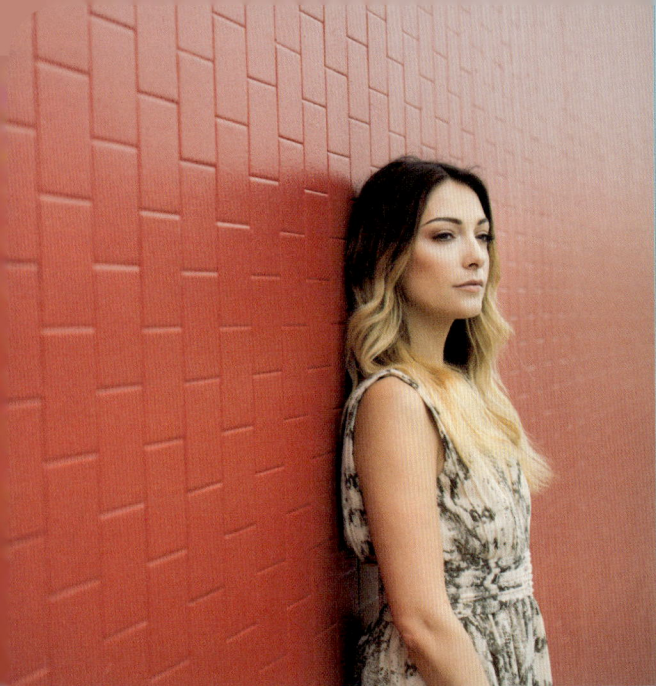

May
18–24
2026

M	T	W	T	F	S	S
				1	2	3
4	5	6	7	8	9	10
11	12	13	14	15	16	17
18	**19**	**20**	**21**	**22**	**23**	**24**
25	26	27	28	29	30	31

CHECK YOUR POSTURE

Hunched sitting and slouchy walking don't just make you look sloppy: Poor posture can slow blood circulation and cause pain or creakiness. It may also be linked to chronic fatigue. Grab a pal and see where you stand by doing this easy posture test:

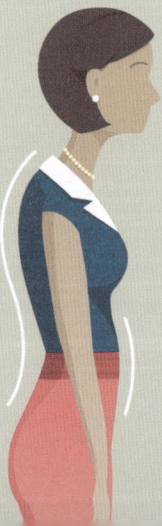

POOR POSTURE

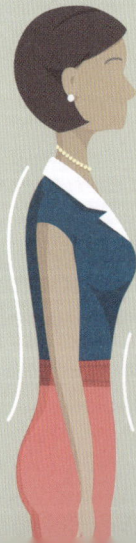

GOOD POSTURE

Try It Now

1. Stand against a wall with your heels planted six inches away from it and the back of your head touching the wall. Be sure your buttocks and both shoulder blades also make contact with the wall.

2. Have someone measure the space between your neck and the wall and also the distance between the wall and the small of your back.

3. If both measurements are two inches or less, your posture is great! Gaps greater than two inches suggest your posture could use some work. Your doctor can give you tips for improving your posture or refer you to a specialist who can.

18 Monday

19 Tuesday

20 Wednesday

21 Thursday

22 Friday

23 Saturday ◑

24 Sunday

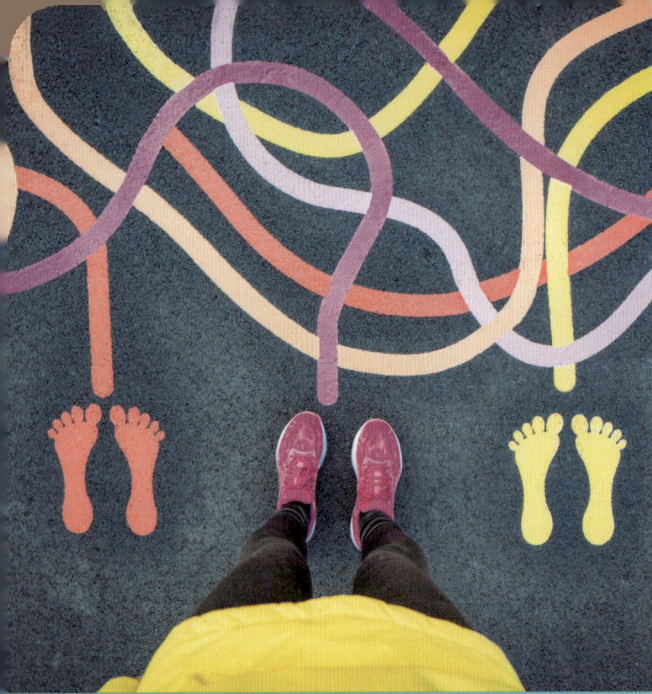

May
25–31
2026

M	T	W	T	F	S	S
				1	2	3
4	5	6	7	8	9	10
11	12	13	14	15	16	17
18	19	20	21	22	23	24
25	26	27	28	29	30	31

CHOOSE THE RIGHT SHOE

If you're inspired to add walking or running to your fitness routine, good for you! Just make sure your feet are equipped with the right shoe. A walker's needs are different than a runner's needs, so the standard design of walking and running shoes differ in important ways. Experts say you should pay close attention to shoe weight, cushioning, and flexibility.

Here's What to Know

In general, running shoes are designed to be more lightweight, but that comes at a cost for walkers who might find that such shoes offer less stability. For example, the cushioning in a running shoe is more localized since runners care most about protecting their foot's base as it continually hits the ground. Likewise, running shoes don't provide the flexibility in the shoe sole that walkers need for the consistent heel-to-toe movement, leaving them vulnerable to damaging the soles of their feet. Whatever you choose, monitor how you feel and replace them after every 300 to 400 miles or every four to six months.

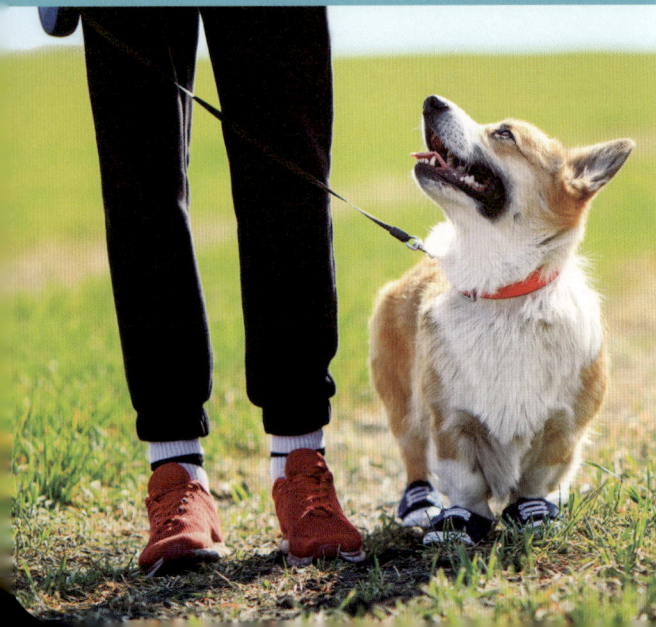

25 Monday Memorial Day

26 Tuesday

27 Wednesday

28 Thursday

29 Friday

30 Saturday

31 Sunday ○

JUNE 2026

MONDAY	TUESDAY	WEDNESDAY	THURSDAY
1	2	3	4
8 ◑	9	10	11
15 ●	16	17	18
22	23	24	25
29 ○	30		

FRIDAY	SATURDAY	SUNDAY
5	6	7
12	13	14 Flag Day
19 Juneteenth	20	21 Father's Day First Day of Summer ◐
26	27	28

MOVE WELL

Check Your SPF Stock. You don't want to get caught without sun protection! Dermatologists recommend smearing on sunscreen with at least SPF 30 about half an hour before heading outdoors and reapplying it every two hours or after being in the water. There are sunblock options to satisfy any sensory need, from lotions to sprays, gels, and even powders.

MAY

M	T	W	T	F	S	S
				1	2	3
4	5	6	7	8	9	10
11	12	13	14	15	16	17
18	19	20	21	22	23	24
25	26	27	28	29	30	31

JULY

M	T	W	T	F	S	S
		1	2	3	4	5
6	7	8	9	10	11	12
13	14	15	16	17	18	19
20	21	22	23	24	25	26
27	28	29	30	31		

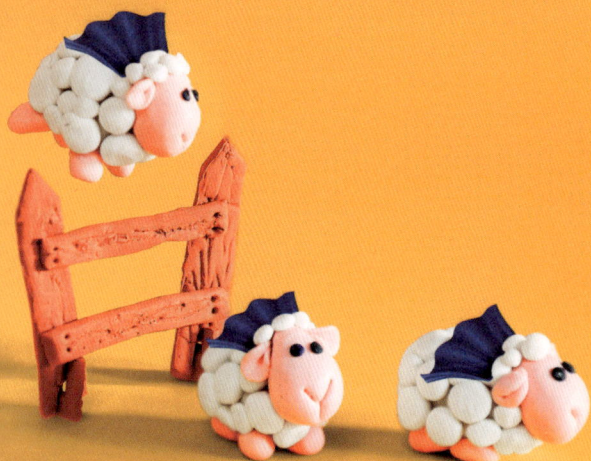

June
1–7
2026

M	T	W	T	F	S	S
1	2	3	4	5	6	7
8	9	10	11	12	13	14
15	16	17	18	19	20	21
22	23	24	25	26	27	28
29	30					

ENJOY BETTER SLEEP

Need another reason to add more exercise to your life? A study published in *BMJ Open* analyzed data from more than 4,300 people between the ages of 39 and 67 over a 10-year period that showed participants who were persistently active (meaning, they exercised for at least an hour a week) were less likely to say that they had trouble falling asleep.

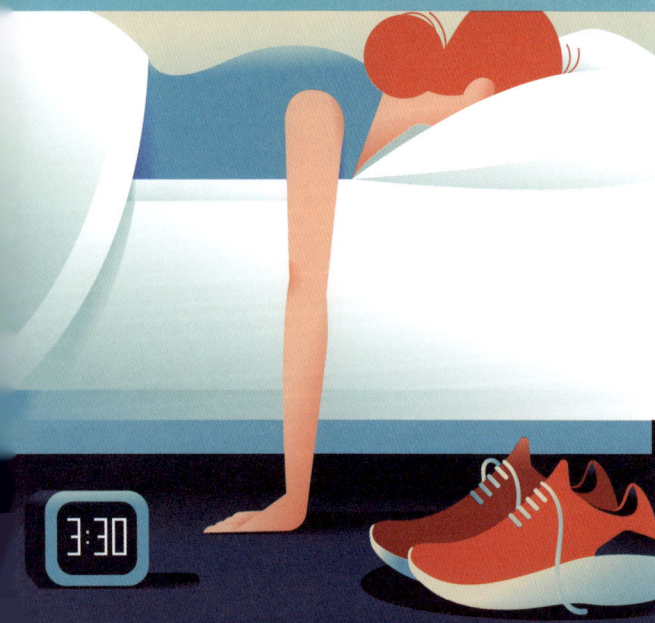

What We Know

Being active can do even more for your sleep health than making you feel wiped, according to behavioral sleep medicine specialist Shelby Harris, Psy.D., a clinical psychologist in private practice in White Plains, New York, and director of sleep health with Sleepopolis. "It helps you relax, sets your body's internal clock, reduces stress, and boosts your mood," she says. It also makes your sleep deeper and more restful, helps you manage your weight, and keeps you healthier overall, she adds.

3:30

1 Monday

2 Tuesday

3 Wednesday

4 Thursday

5 Friday

6 Saturday

7 Sunday

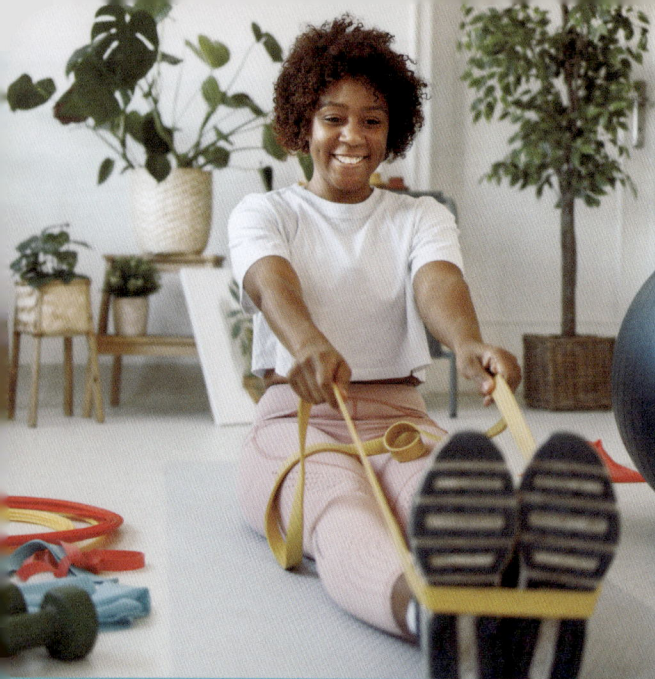

June
8–14
2026

M	T	W	T	F	S	S
1	2	3	4	5	6	7
8	9	10	11	12	13	14
15	16	17	18	19	20	21
22	23	24	25	26	27	28
29	30					

TRY RESISTANCE BANDS

Feeling overwhelmed by fitness can lead to a cycle of adopting, dropping, and then struggling to readopt extreme or unsustainable exercise plans. This in turn can lead to guilt over not reaching your goals and a mindset that's not conducive to success. Instead, why not focus on some exercise equipment that can set you up for best results?

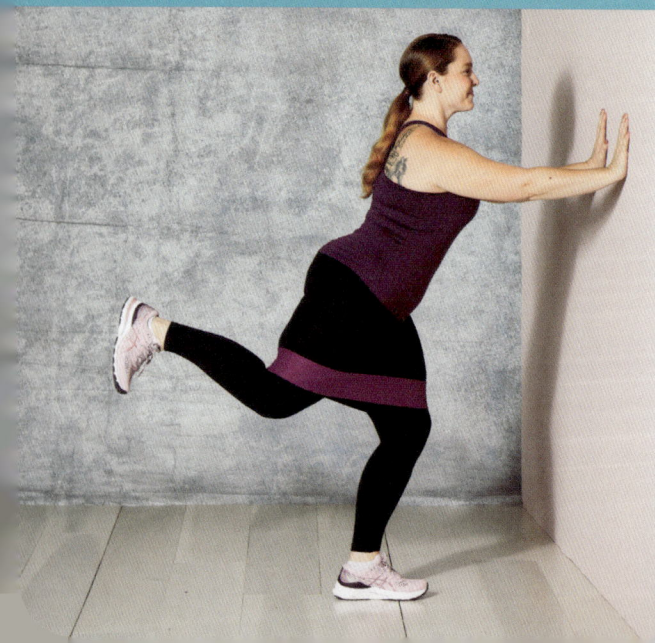

Why It Works

Resistance bands are your secret weapon in your exercise equipment arsenal: They're inexpensive and portable, so they eliminate the need for a bunch of different dumbbells. Plus, they're made from ultra-stretchy materials like rubber and latex and can help you execute moves with better form through building body awareness.

Look for a combination package that includes a variety of resistance weights (light, medium, and hard). Having various weights gives you flexibility to swap what you're using if you find the exercise is too easy (or too difficult). Some bands also have handles on them, which some people find easier to use.

8 Monday ◑

9 Tuesday

10 Wednesday

11 Thursday

12 Friday

13 Saturday

14 Sunday Flag Day

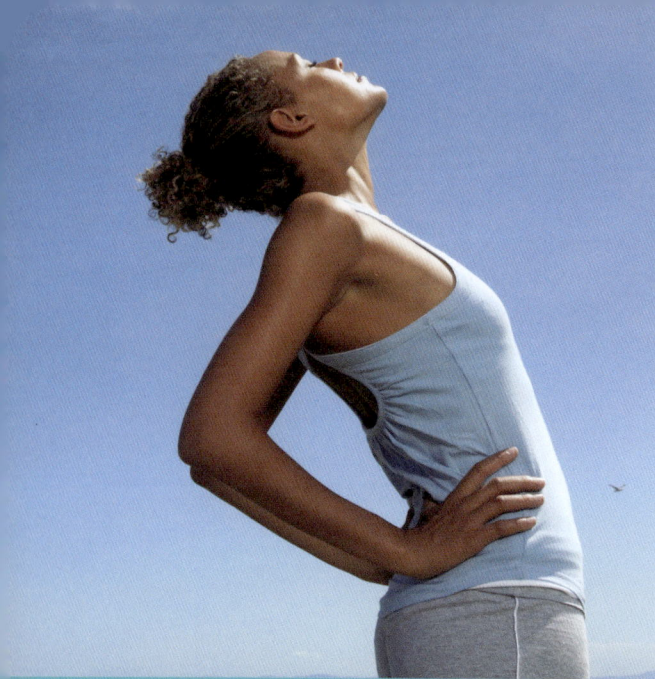

June 15–21

2026

M	T	W	T	F	S	S
1	2	3	4	5	6	7
8	9	10	11	12	13	14
15	16	17	18	19	20	21
22	23	24	25	26	27	28
29	30					

CONSIDER SOMATIC EXERCISES

Unlike cardio and weightlifting routines, somatic exercise is a movement therapy that involves performing movement for the sake of movement, following what feels supportive to your body, versus following the lead of an instructor and using your mind to imitate the instructor's movement. It can be very calming!

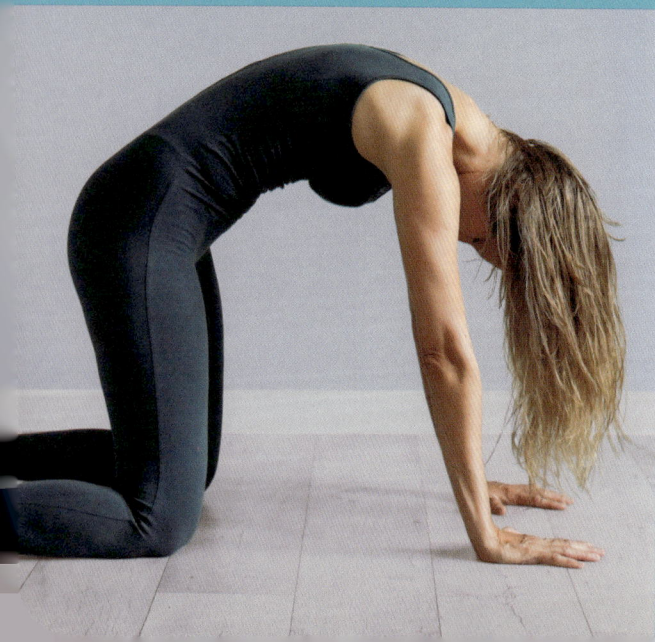

Try It Now

Research on somatic exercise as a treatment for trauma and anxiety is limited, and more is warranted to determine its potential. However, a 2021 review found preliminary evidence that somatic exercise may be an effective treatment for PSTD-related symptoms and may also be useful in the treatment of other disorders. Here are a few simple ones to try:

Heel drops. Slowly raise yourself up onto your toes and then drop back onto your heels.

Wave breathing. Inhale and create an arch in your back. Exhale and curl forward.

Sway. Sway from side to side. Breathe and relax.

15 Monday ●

16 Tuesday

17 Wednesday

18 Thursday

19 Friday Juneteenth

20 Saturday

21 Sunday ◑ Father's Day
First Day of Summer

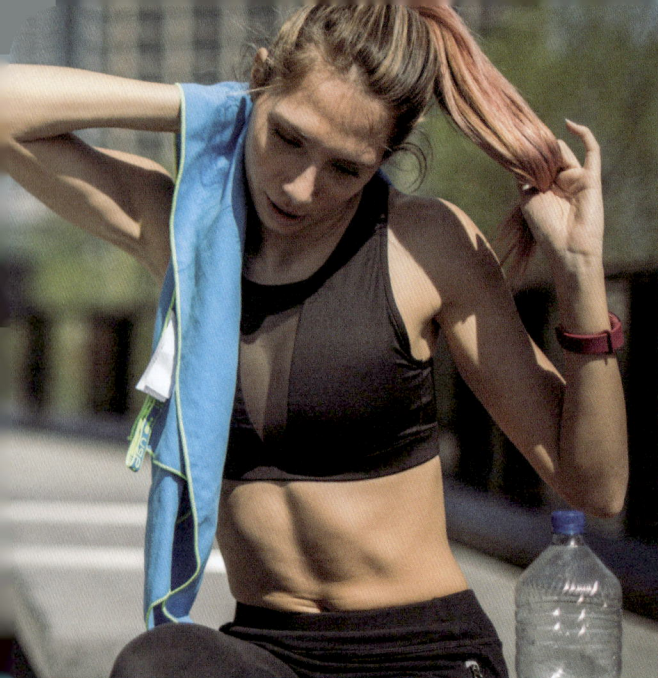

June
22–28
2026

M	T	W	T	F	S	S
1	2	3	4	5	6	7
8	9	10	11	12	13	14
15	16	17	18	19	20	21
22	**23**	**24**	**25**	**26**	**27**	**28**
29	30					

BEAT THE HEAT

Whenever you enjoy an outdoor workout in warm weather, keeping cool in the heat is essential. Cooling towels to the rescue! Unlike regular towels, cooling towels are designed to offer immediate relief. They bring a cooling sensation to your skin, helping you stay comfortable and avoid overheating, reducing the risk of heat exhaustion and heatstroke.

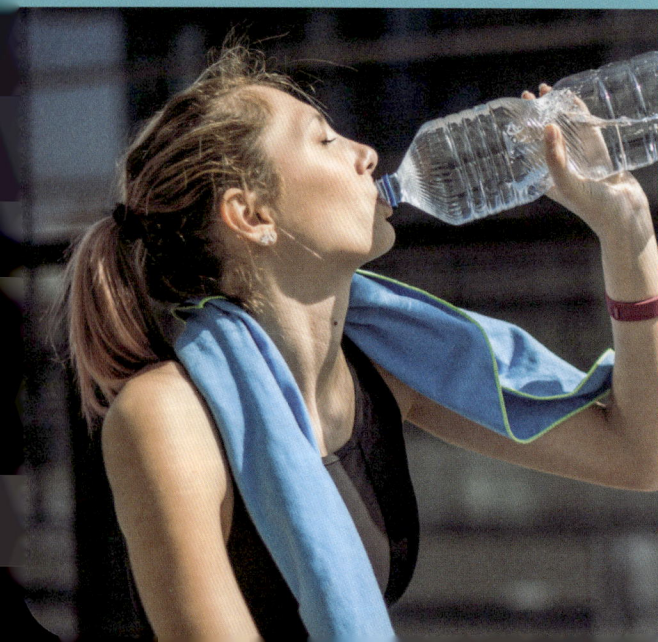

What to Do

To use a cooling towel to boost your other hydration efforts, just wet it with water, wring it out, and snap it a few times. Then apply it to the area in need of relief (around your neck is ideal for full-body cooling). "When the cooling towel is placed on your skin, it draws the heat away from your body as the water evaporates" says Patricia Greaves, C.P.T., a corrective exercise specialist and nutrition coach and the founder of StrongHer Personal Training. Most cooling towels are made from high-tech cooling fabrics that are designed to act like sponges and can hold more water for longer periods without feeling heavy or transferring moisture to your clothing.

22 Monday

23 Tuesday

24 Wednesday

25 Thursday

26 Friday

27 Saturday

28 Sunday

SUMMER
STRESS LESS ABOUT
FOOD

When you think about how intertwined food and cognitive health are, it's no surprise that what you eat also impacts mental health—in a couple of ways. For one, "nutrition plays a direct role in hormone and neurotransmitter synthesis, influencing mood-regulating chemicals like serotonin, dopamine, and norepinephrine," explains Laura Iu, C.D.N., a registered dietitian in New York City.

And sometimes food can boost your mood simply because of how it makes you feel—through tastes, textures, or nostalgia. "Comfort foods have gotten a bad rap for being 'unhealthy,' but enjoying comfort food from time to time is important for everyone," says Judy Ho, Ph.D., a neuropsychologist and the author of *The New Rules of Attachment*. This season we'll help you know which foods to choose to help your body better manage stress, as well as ways to find your calm and improve your mindset during mealtime.

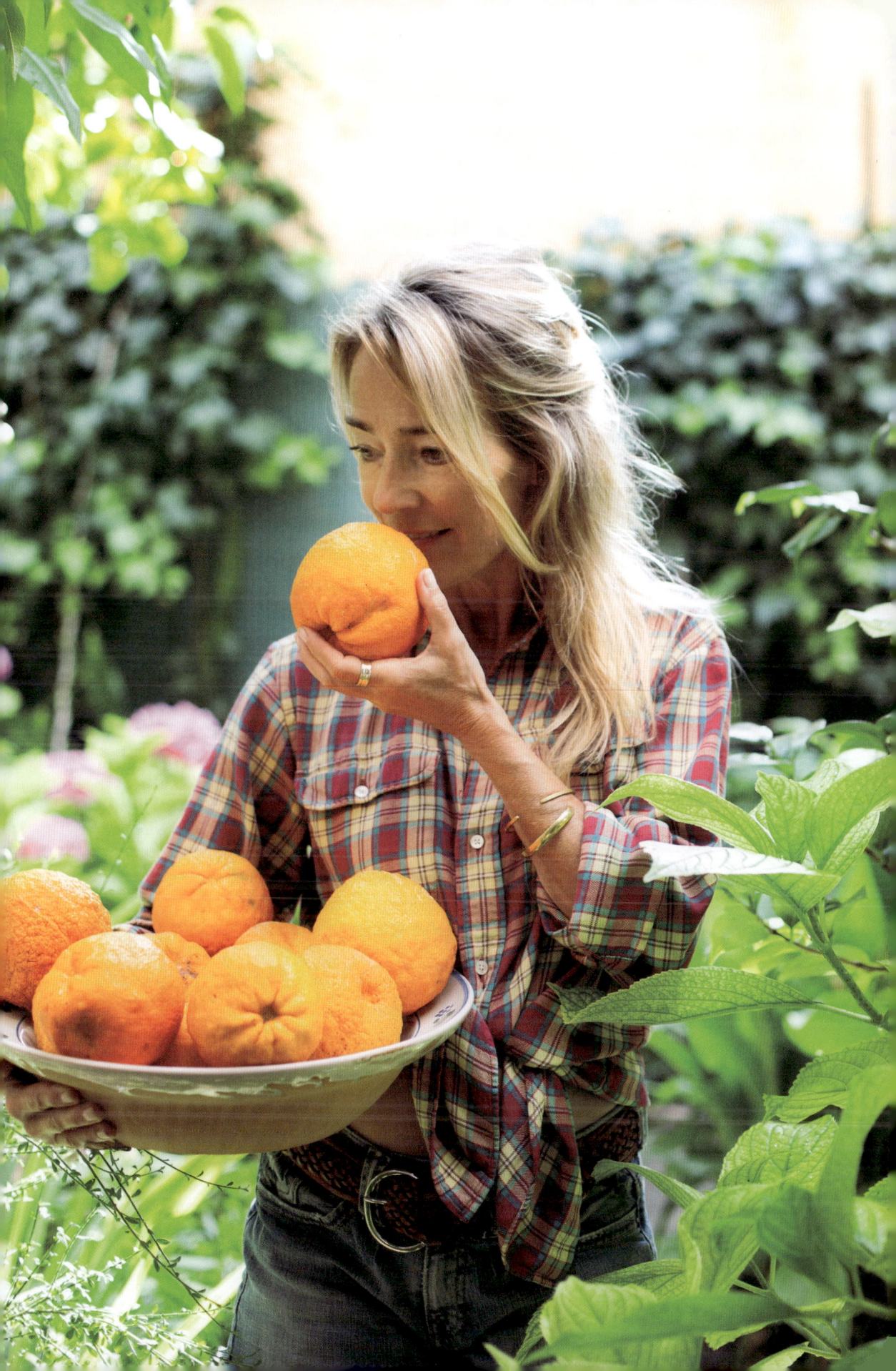

Choose Good Mood Foods

Nobody is upbeat 24/7. But knowing what helps you get back to baseline when you're down is essential for head-to-toe health, as consistently poor mental health can raise your risk for chronic diseases. Your anytime mood boosters: the right foods.

"Specific nutrients play a direct role in hormone and neurotransmitter synthesis, influencing mood-regulating chemicals like serotonin and dopamine," says Iu. Plus, certain foods simply make you feel happy when you eat them, says Ho. Incorporating these foods into your day may just lift your spirits:

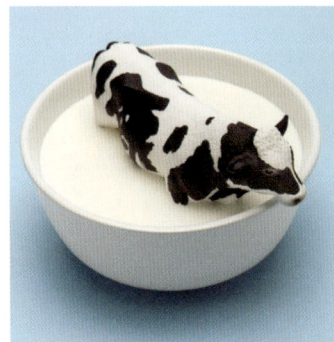

Dairy Milk, cheese, and yogurt could contribute to reducing and preventing depressive symptoms. "A recent large study found that as calcium intake increased, symptoms of depression decreased," says Ho. "Vitamin D may also help improve mood by elevating serotonin levels in the brain."

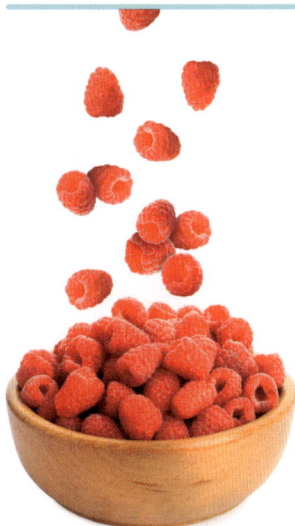

Dark Chocolate

It's lower in sugar than milk chocolate, which means less risk of an energy crash, and it contains antioxidants that tend to boost positive emotions, says Ho.

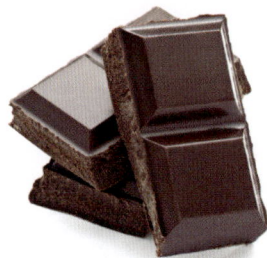

Raspberries

These sweet guys get their vibrancy from anthocyanins, antioxidants with an anti-inflammatory effect, says Iu. This is helpful, as inflammation may increase the risk of mood and psychiatric disorders, research shows. One study has even suggested that higher anthocyanin intake is associated with fewer depression symptoms.

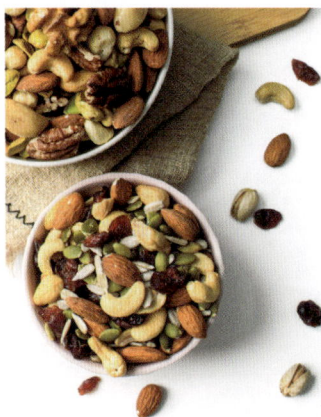

Nuts and Seeds

These are a great source of omega-3s, which help keep stress hormones like cortisol and adrenaline under control, explains Ho. Olive oil and avocado are also rich in omega-3s.

Turkey

"Tryptophan is a nutrient that I consider crucial for good mental health, as it helps synthesize serotonin in the brain, which can help improve mood," Iu explains. Turkey contains tryptophan and tyrosine, another amino acid that helps the brain make and regulate dopamine, the pleasure hormone.

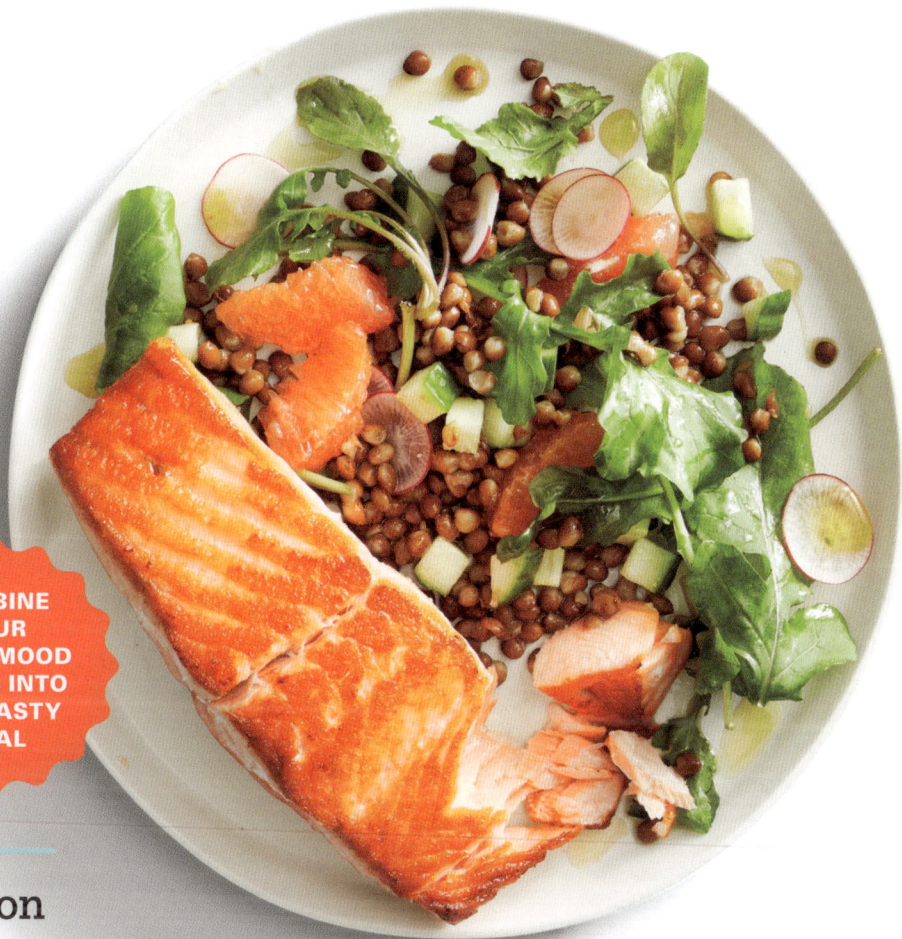

COMBINE YOUR GOOD-MOOD FOODS INTO ONE TASTY MEAL

Salmon

It delivers healthy fats and vitamin D, two essentials for managing stress, anxiety, and depression. Low levels of the "sunshine vitamin" have been associated with increased risk of depression and anxiety, Iu says, and fat impacts how mood-related chemicals and hormones function.

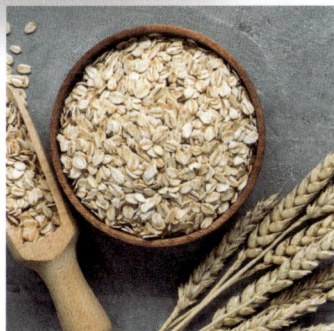

Lentils
B vitamins are biggies for good mental health and cognitive function, says Iu—and legumes like lentils are a great source. "Low levels of folate have been associated with increased risk of depression and anxiety," she adds. Lentils also have fiber to support balanced blood sugar levels and, in turn, mood.

Oats
Whole grains such as oats are complex carbs, and they help regulate blood sugar for a more stable mood; they also provide B vitamins, which contribute to the production of serotonin, a brain chemical that elicits feelings of relaxation and wellness, says Ho.

Cocoa
Beyond flavonols, which tame inflammation, cocoa has antioxidants "which tend to induce feelings of relaxation and support healthy blood pressure," Ho says. And chocolate is a comfort food for many, which can aid in its mood-steadying abilities, she adds.

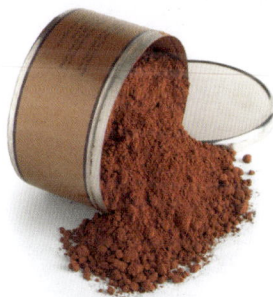

Elevate Your Mental Health at Mealtimes

Mindfulness has been shown to be a wonderful antidote to stress and anxiety, which can make a big difference in how physically and mentally vibrant you feel. When you slow down and focus on enjoying your food (noticing taste, texture, and smell) instead of shoveling it in or chowing down as you scroll social media, you give yourself a chance to reset each time you eat, whether it's a meal or a protein bar. Follow these steps:

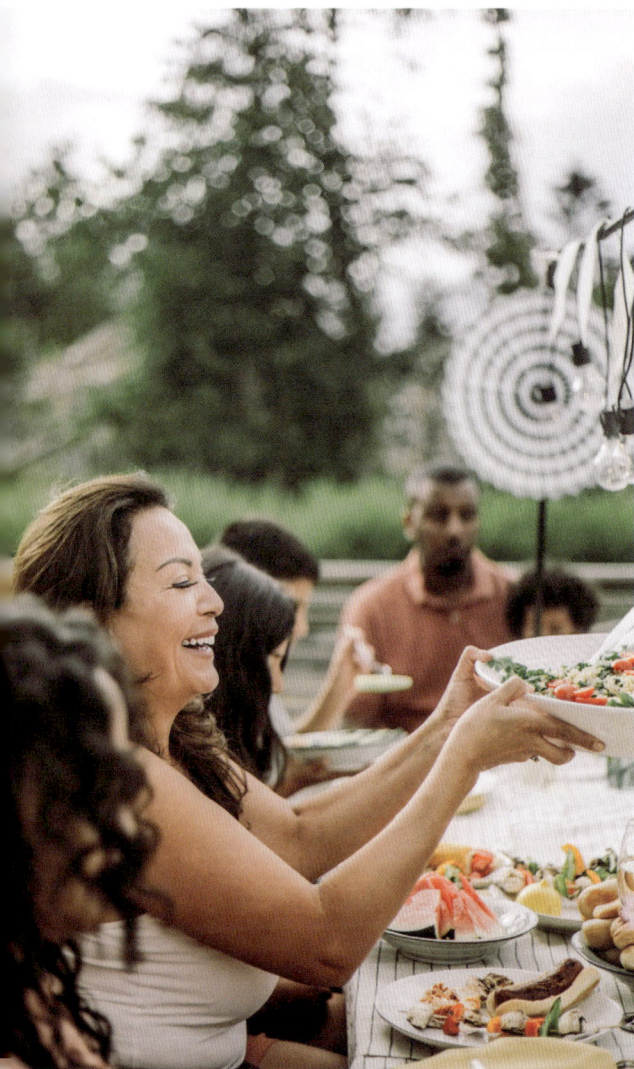

BEFORE YOU SIT... Assess how you feel. Being slightly hungry is OK, but anything more extreme can make it hard to pump the brakes and be mindful. Make a mental commitment to enjoying balanced meals throughout the day so that at mealtimes you will have an appetite but won't be ravenous.

ONCE SEATED... Start with gratitude. Take a minute or two to pause and appreciate the food in front of you. Focus on being grateful for your body as well as this meal and everything and everyone involved in preparing it. Are you sharing this eating experience with friends or family members? Spend a moment reflecting on and expressing appreciation for them too.

AT FIRST BITE... Utilize your senses right off the bat. Pay attention to different flavors and aromas. How does the food sound when you chew it? Does it feel crunchy or smooth? Do the flavors or textures change throughout the meal? These are examples of questions you can ask yourself during a mindful eating experience.

AS YOU NOSH... Take time to chew your food, notice its flavor, and savor each bite. This should help you slow your eating pace, but if you find that you're still going fast, try to set your fork down after every few bites. It takes about 20 minutes for your stomach to signal to your brain that it's full.

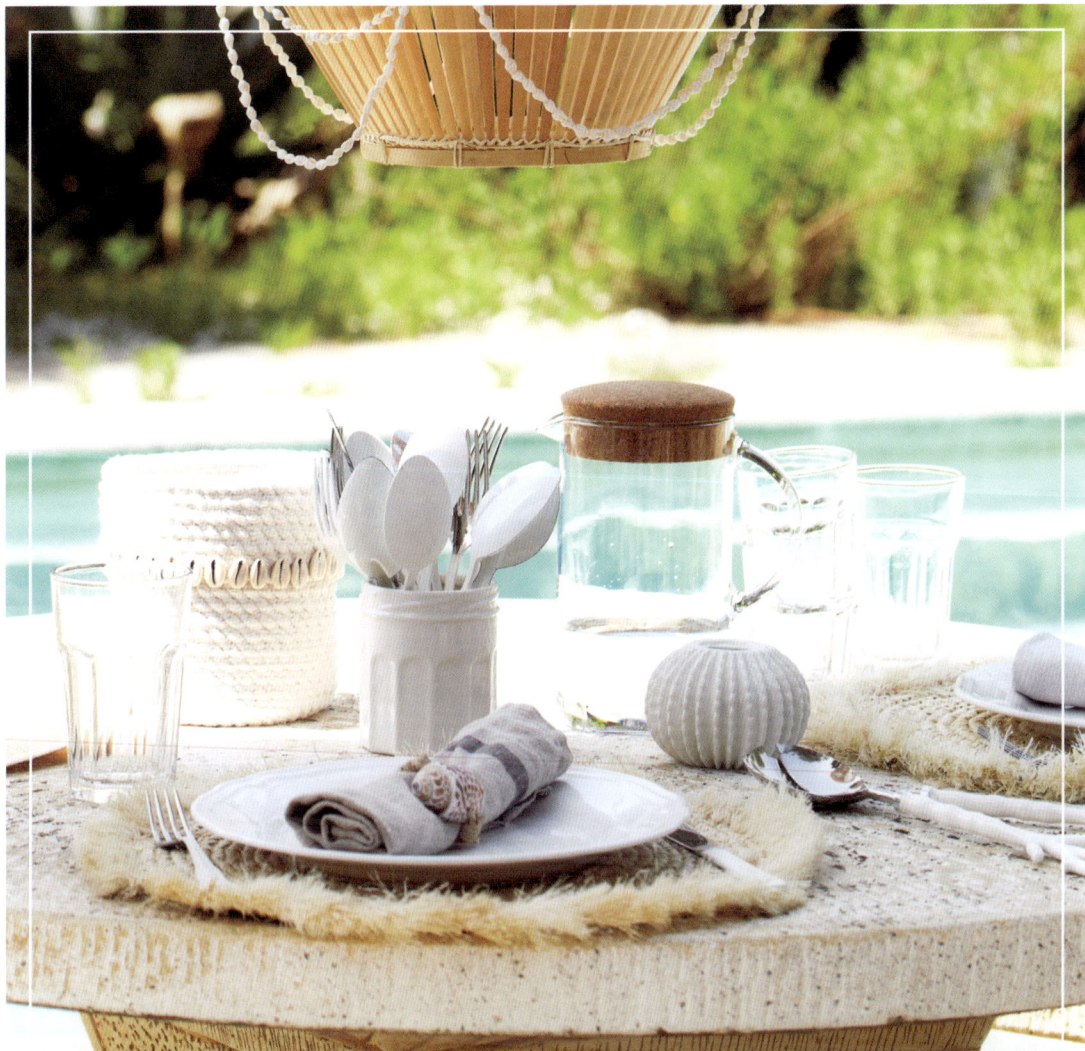

Make Mindful Eating Even Easier

Place phones and other electronics in a basket at the beginning of mealtime to minimize distractions.

• Turn off the TV and anything else that may shift your focus away from the activity at hand: eating.

• Create a nice decorative table-scape or use dishware that brings you joy to set the mood.

• Choose foods you like that are easy to prepare, and enjoy your meal with a glass of plain or sparkling water with lemon or lime slices instead of a sugary drink or an alcoholic one.

• Take a relaxing postmeal walk, journal about your thoughts, or cue up an inspiring dishwashing playlist to further boost your satisfaction.

JULY 2026

MONDAY	TUESDAY	WEDNESDAY	THURSDAY
		1	2
6	7 ◑	8	9
13	14 ●	15	16
20	21 ◐	22	23
27	28	29 ○	30

FRIDAY	SATURDAY	SUNDAY
3	4 Independence Day	5
10	11	12
17	18	19
24	25	26
31		

EAT WELL

Make a "No Food Waste" Plan. Then start putting it into action this month! Reduce the stress you feel when you need to toss leftovers before they go bad. Learn how to use more of various foods (turn carrot tops into pesto, for instance, and use leaves and stems of herbs). Make a grocery list to avoid overbuying. And check out smartphone apps that let you "rescue" food headed for the curb.

JUNE

M	T	W	T	F	S	S
1	2	3	4	5	6	7
8	9	10	11	12	13	14
15	16	17	18	19	20	21
22	23	24	25	26	27	28
29	30					

AUGUST

M	T	W	T	F	S	S
					1	2
3	4	5	6	7	8	9
10	11	12	13	14	15	16
17	18	19	20	21	22	23
24	25	26	27	28	29	30
31						

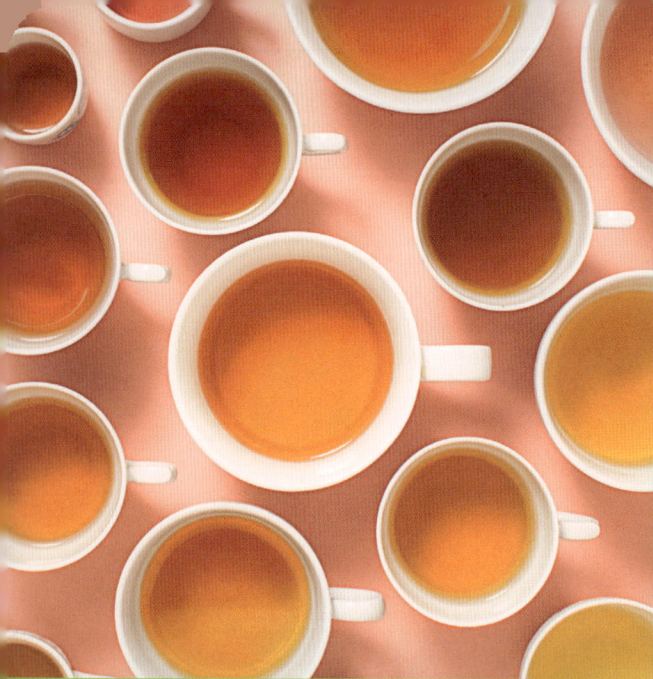

June 29– July 5

2026

M	T	W	T	F	S	S
29	30	1	2	3	4	5
6	7	8	9	10	11	12
13	14	15	16	17	18	19
20	21	22	23	24	25	26
27	28	29	30	31		

SHARPEN YOUR FOCUS

Tea is one of the most consumed beverages in the world other than water, making it a major part of many people's lives. While it's a reliable mood booster given that it's warm, comforting, tastes good, and you can get it for a low price just about anywhere, there are real health benefits of black tea to consider the next time you brew a cup.

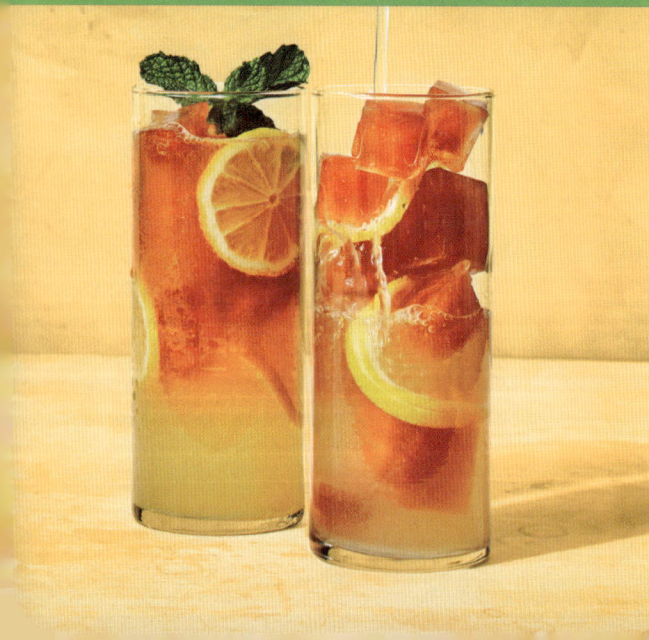

Why It Works

The caffeine in black tea can increase your focus and energy level while helping you avoid that eye-twitching, overcaffeinated feeling you can get from drinking coffee. A cup of brewed tea has from a quarter to half the amount of caffeine as a cup of coffee, so it's great for people who want extra support without an overly stimulating sip, says integrative dietitian Robin Foroutan, R.D.N. "Because tea has caffeine along with L-theanine, a compound that helps your body regulate the calming neurotransmitters, black tea can give you a more balanced boost," she adds.

29 Monday

30 Tuesday

1 Wednesday

2 Thursday

3 Friday

4 Saturday Independence Day

5 Sunday

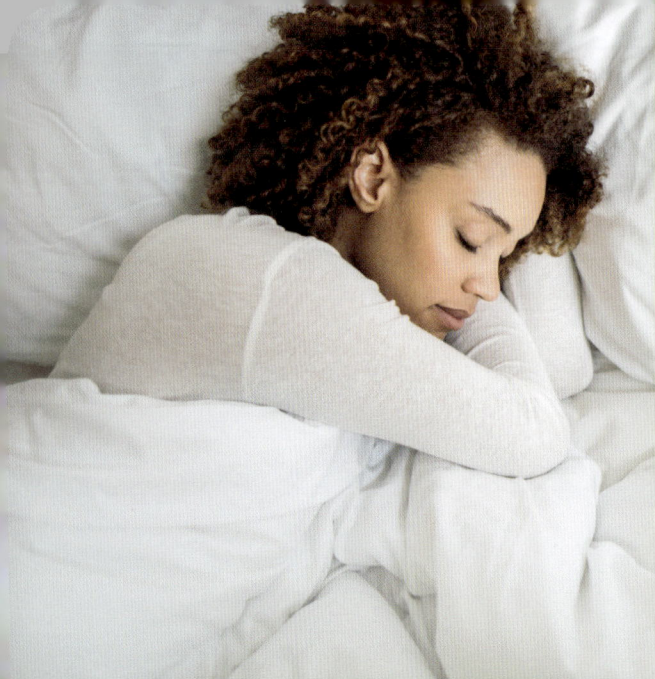

July
6–12
2026

M	T	W	T	F	S	S
			1	2	3	4	5
6	7	8	9	10	11	12
13	14	15	16	17	18	19
20	21	22	23	24	25	26
27	28	29	30	31		

ENJOY BREAKFAST BEFORE BED

Ever say good night and then have your stomach enter the conversation with a loud grumbling that means "Feed me"? Don't let it stress you out. Contrary to what you might have heard about pre-bed snacking messing with sleep, the right bed-time snack can actually help summon zzz's—or at least satisfy your peck-ishness so you can nod off.

Try It Now

The right combination of nutrients is key to making the best choice, and a bowl of cereal can be a perfect and easy option. Carbohydrates in whole-grain cereal help you fall asleep, and protein-rich milk helps you stay asleep, says Jaclyn London, M.S., R.D., a New York City–based registered dietitian and podcast host and the author of *Dressing on the Side (and Other Diet Myths Debunked)*. "Milk is chock-full of calcium and magnesium, which help you produce melatonin, the hormone respon-sible for sleep regulation," London adds. Choose a low-sugar cereal with 4 grams or less of the sweet stuff, and opt for lowfat or nonfat milk.

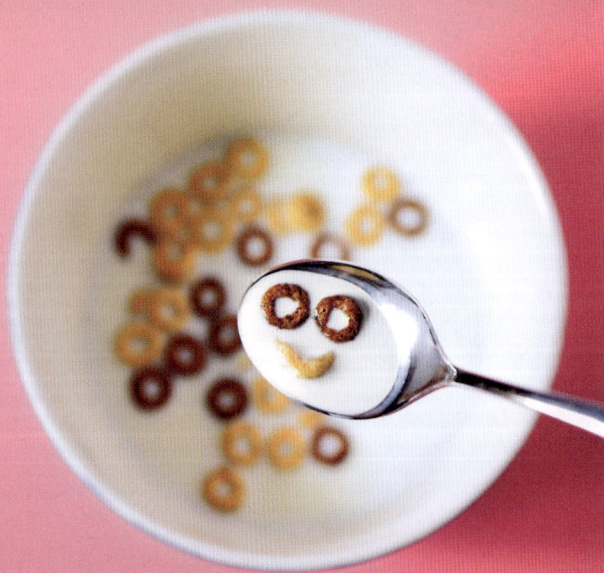

6 Monday

7 Tuesday ◑

8 Wednesday

9 Thursday

10 Friday

11 Saturday

12 Sunday

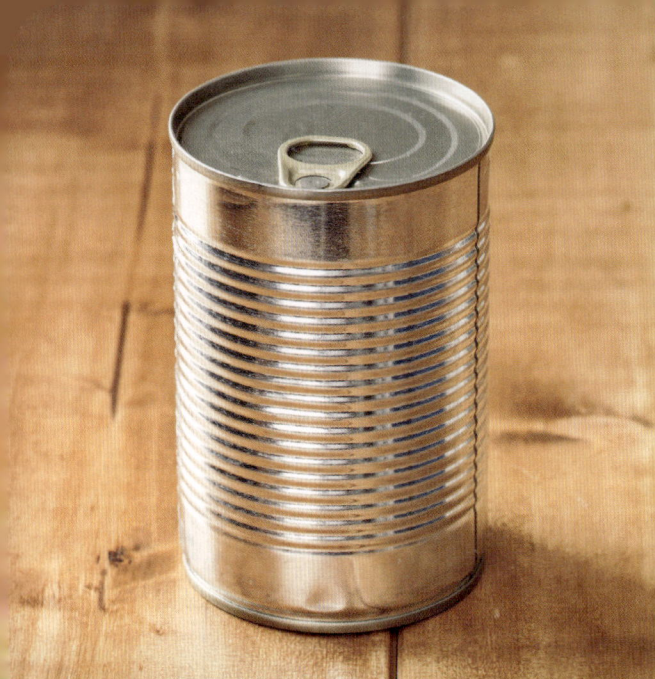

July
13–19
2026

M	T	W	T	F	S	S
		1	2	3	4	5
6	7	8	9	10	11	12
13	14	15	16	17	18	19
20	21	22	23	24	25	26
27	28	29	30	31		

PERK UP YOUR PANTRY

Do you buy the same things on every supermarket run? Use your habitual nature to make wise eating a little easier and less stressful: Grab a variety of canned foods on each trip and keep them on hand so you'll always have nutritious staples with which to create a balanced meal, even on your most tiring days.

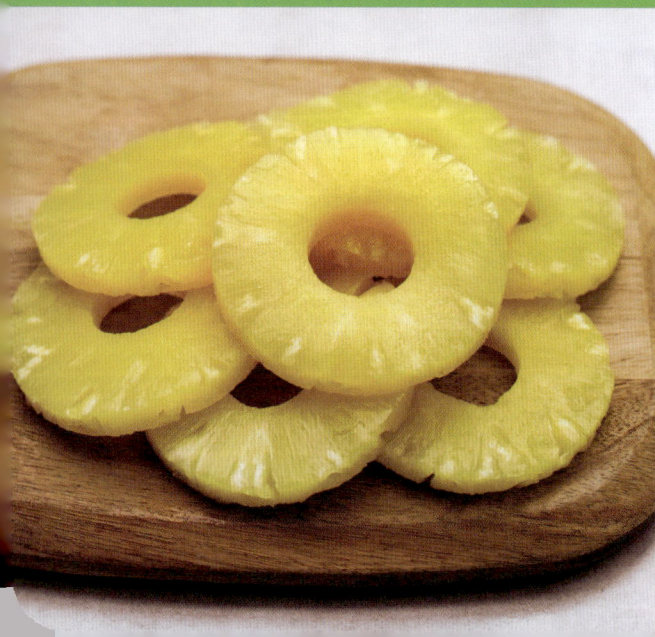

What to Do

Stefani Sassos, M.S., R.D.N., the Good Housekeeping Institute's nutrition director, recommends canned produce or beans that (ideally) contain only the food itself. Choose foods low in sodium and go for fruit in water or its own juice. Kickstart your pantry makeover with these canned essentials:

- Hearts of palm are a source of vitamin B6, which plays a role in immune and nervous system function.
- Cannellini beans provide fiber and plant-based protein to keep blood sugar (and mood) stable.
- Pineapple contains bromelain, an enzyme that fights inflammation and improves digestion.

13 Monday

14 Tuesday ●

15 Wednesday

16 Thursday

17 Friday

18 Saturday

19 Sunday

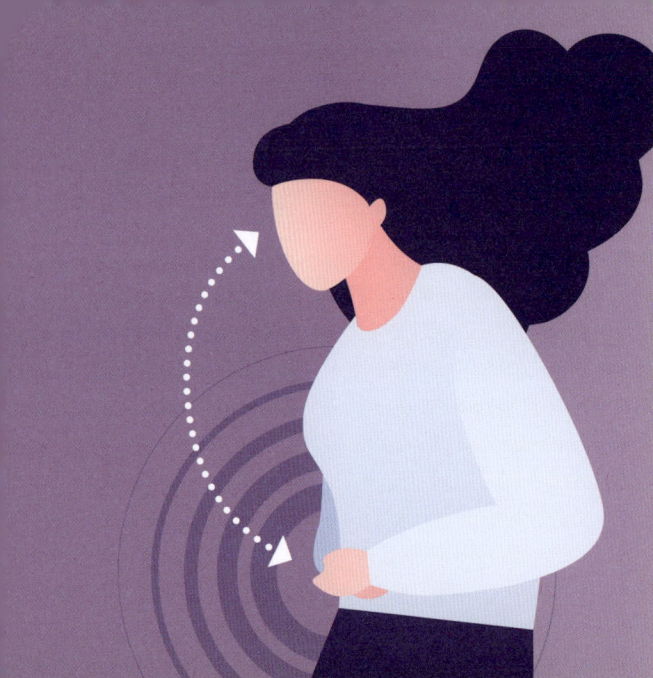

July
20–26
2026

M	T	W	T	F	S	S
		1	2	3	4	5
6	7	8	9	10	11	12
13	14	15	16	17	18	19
20	**21**	**22**	**23**	**24**	**25**	**26**
27	28	29	30	31		

THINK ABOUT THE BRAIN IN YOUR GUT

The brain in your head sends signals to your body about almost everything you feel, including emotions and pain, and many of those signals travel to your digestive tract. In fact, your gut and your brain are more intimately connected than any other body systems, thanks to the large number of nerve cells in the intestines.

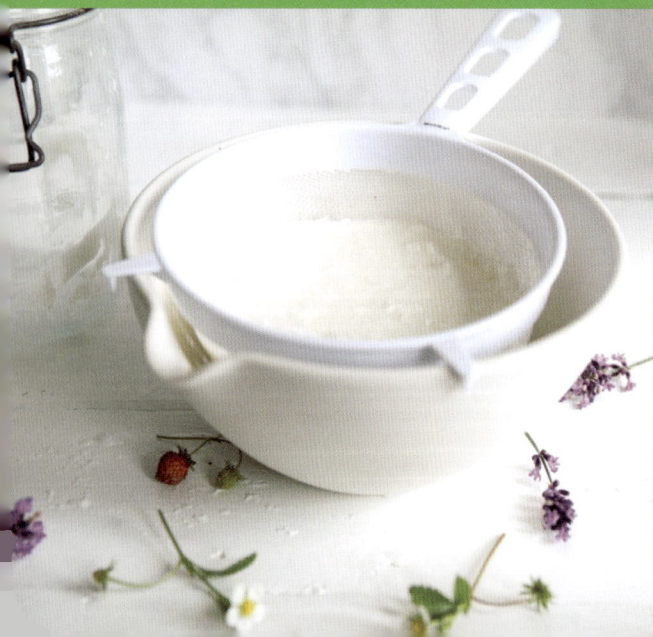

What We Know

The vagus nerve, which goes from the brain down to the gut and beyond, is the main superhighway for this information exchange. Chatter along the gut-brain axis influences digestion as well as pain sensitivity, cognitive function, and the immune system. A large study found that people with severe irritable bowel syndrome (IBS) had twice the rates of depression and anxiety of people without IBS.

Some strategies to improve the health of your gut-brain axis include snacking on fermented foods such as kefir and yogurt and stimulating your vagus nerve with yoga, meditation, or slow and controlled breathing.

20 Monday

21 Tuesday ◑

22 Wednesday

23 Thursday

24 Friday

25 Saturday

26 Sunday

AUGUST 2026

MONDAY	TUESDAY	WEDNESDAY	THURSDAY
3	4	5	6 ◗
10	11	12 ●	13
17	18	19	20 ◐
24	25	26	27
31			

FRIDAY	SATURDAY	SUNDAY
	1	2
7	8	9
14	15	16
21	22	23
28	29	30

EAT WELL

Pick Up a Beach Read. What are you feeding your mind this month? Getting lost in a good book is a great way to spend a leisurely day or a breezy evening; it also benefits your brain and can help ease stress. Why not embrace the season's slow pace by diving into a novel with a summery setting, or another easy read?

JULY

M	T	W	T	F	S	S
	1	2	3	4	5	
6	7	8	9	10	11	12
13	14	15	16	17	18	19
20	21	22	23	24	25	26
27	28	29	30	31		

SEPTEMBER

M	T	W	T	F	S	S
	1	2	3	4	5	6
7	8	9	10	11	12	13
14	15	16	17	18	19	20
21	22	23	24	25	26	27
28	29	30				

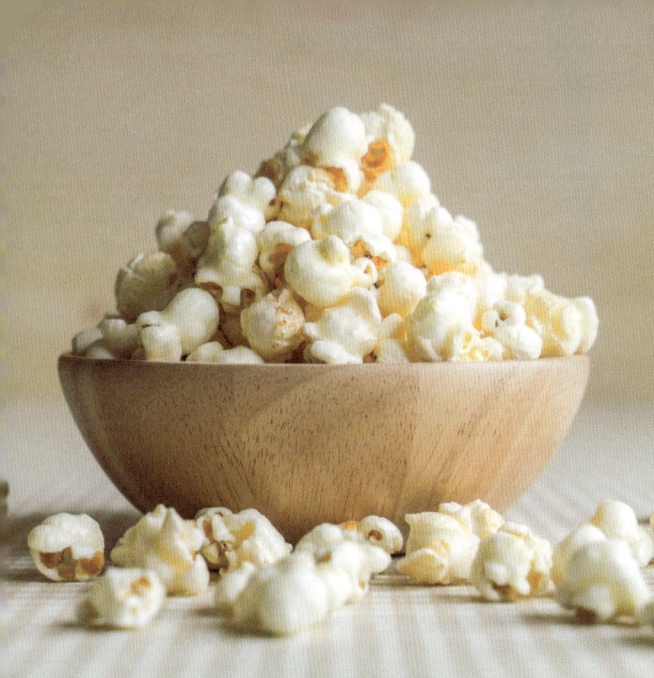

July 27–
August 2
2026

M	T	W	T	F	S	S
27	28	29	30	31	1	2
3	4	5	6	7	8	9
10	11	12	13	14	15	16
17	18	19	20	21	22	23
24	25	26	27	28	29	30
31						

SNACK SMARTER

"I'm a big fan of snacking," says Jaclyn London, R.D., a nutrition consultant and podcast host and the author of *Dressing on the Side (and Other Diet Myths Debunked)*. "Snacks that involve smaller portions of intentional, nutrient-dense combos keep up our energy levels." Use London's smart snacking guidelines, customizing them to your lifestyle.

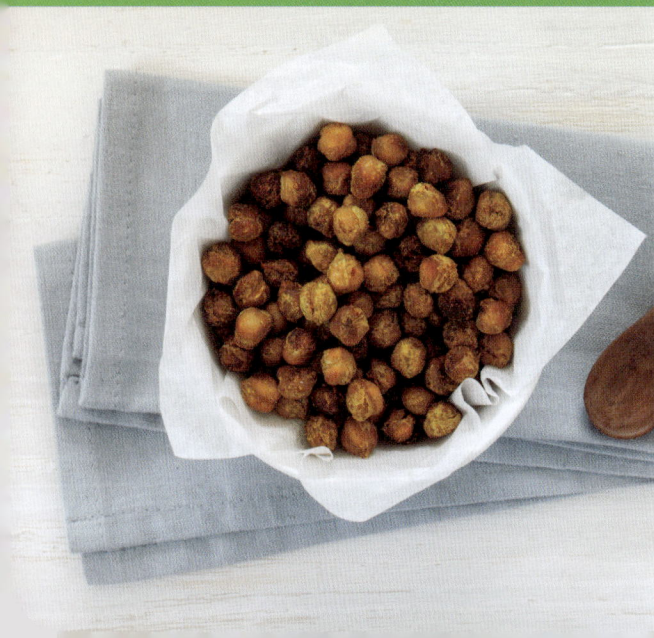

Try It Now

Eat a meal or snack every three to four hours. This schedule supports steady energy and helps you avoid being ravenous going into your next meal.

Make sure your snack contains the satiety trifecta: protein, fiber, and healthy fat. This nutritional equation stabilizes blood sugar to keep your energy and mood even and let you remain full.

Create a snack-sperience. Snacks that are "crunchable and poppable" are easy to differentiate from meals. "I love air-popped popcorn, roasted chickpeas, and frozen grapes," London says.

27 Monday

28 Tuesday

29 Wednesday ○

30 Thursday

31 Friday

1 Saturday

2 Sunday

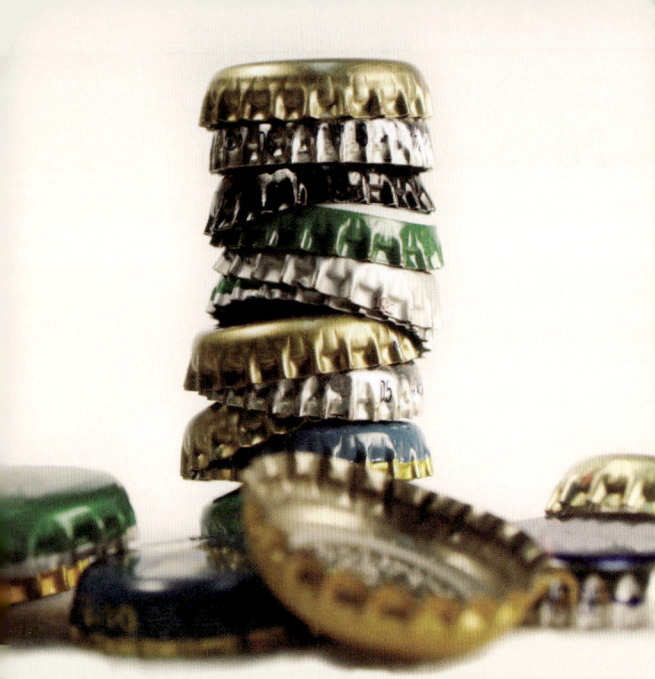

August
3–9
2026

M	T	W	T	F	S	S
					1	2
3	4	5	6	7	8	9
10	11	12	13	14	15	16
17	18	19	20	21	22	23
24	25	26	27	28	29	30
31						

RETHINK DRINKING

Drinking too much has long been associated with depression and anxiety, digestive issues, memory problems, and lowered immunity. It also leads to disinhibition, which can trigger violent or risky behavior. An estimated 28.8 million U.S. adults have alcohol use disorder (AUD), a condition that makes it difficult to stop or control drinking.

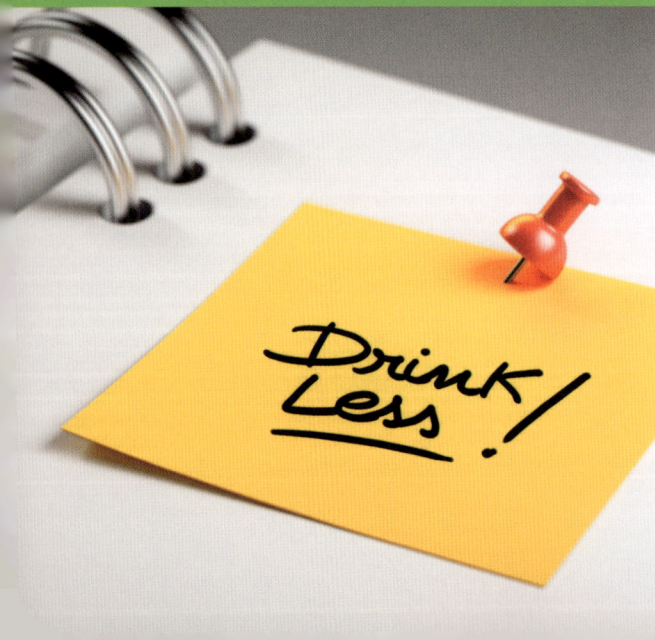

Here's What to Do

Instead of the vague "Cut back," set a limit like "No more than three drinks in a week." Write down your goals so they won't be subject to change and so you can read them on days when you may feel tempted to drink more, says Sergio Muriel, a certified addiction professional and the chief operating officer of Diamond Behavioral Health in Palm Beach, FL. Also, make sure you consider which people or situations ignite the urge to drink. Then fill your time with more supportive people and healthier activities instead. If you struggle to cut back, don't hesitate to get help through therapy or rehab.

3 Monday

4 Tuesday

5 Wednesday

6 Thursday ◑

7 Friday

8 Saturday

9 Sunday

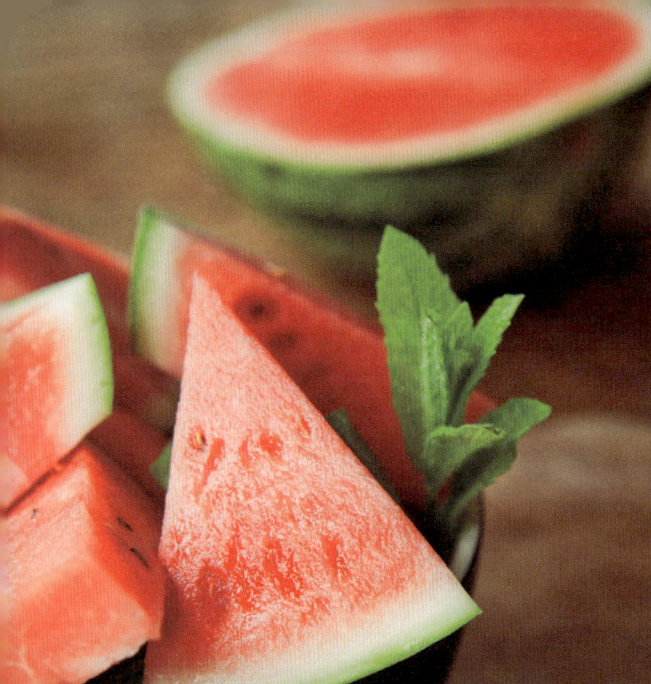

August
10–16
2026

M	T	W	T	F	S	S
					1	2
3	4	5	6	7	8	9
10	11	12	13	14	15	16
17	18	19	20	21	22	23
24	25	26	27	28	29	30
31						

ENJOY AN EASY DESSERT

Here's a refreshing treat to enjoy during the dog days of summer. To serve, simply use a fork to scrape the watermelon mixture and create large flakes, and then transfer to bowls or glasses. Top with sparkling water if desired, and serve with mint.

Try This Now
WATERMELON-MINT GRANITA

Active 15 min. | **Total** 4 hr. 15 min.
SERVES 4 TO 6

2	lbs cubed watermelon		1	tsp grated lime zest, plus 2 Tbsp lime juice
⅓	cup fresh mint leaves, plus more for serving			Kosher salt

1. In blender, puree watermelon, mint, lime zest and juice, and a pinch of salt until smooth.

2. Transfer mixture to 8- by 8-in. metal baking pan and freeze until firm, 3 to 4 hr.

PER SERVING: 57 cal, 1 g pro, 19 g carb, 2 g fiber, 16.5 g sugars, (0 g added sugars), 0 g fat (0 g sat fat), 0 mg chol, 32 mg sodium

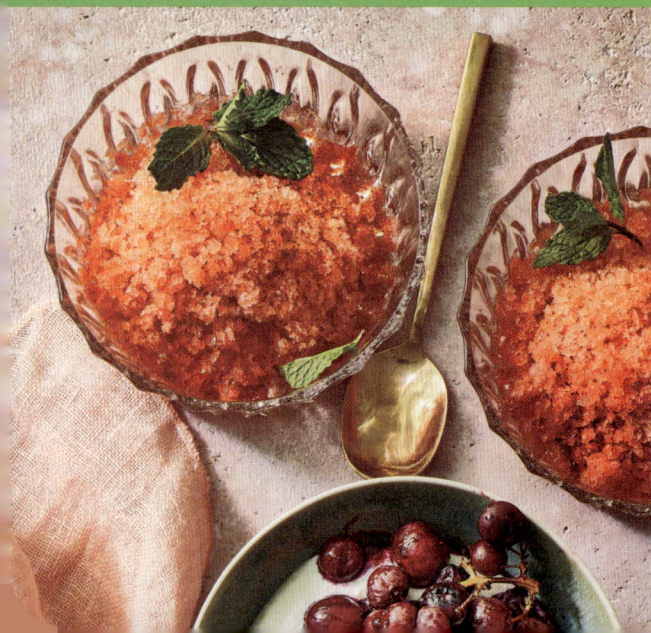

10 Monday

11 Tuesday

12 Wednesday ●

13 Thursday

14 Friday

15 Saturday

16 Sunday

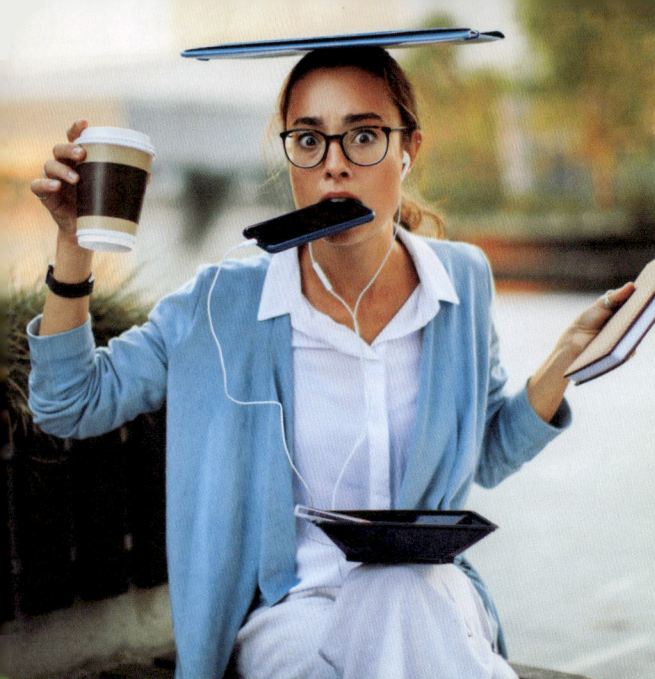

August
17–23
2026

M	T	W	T	F	S	S
					1	2
3	4	5	6	7	8	9
10	11	12	13	14	15	16
17	**18**	**19**	**20**	**21**	**22**	**23**
24	25	26	27	28	29	30
31						

STOP STRESS EATING

Stress eating involves turning to food when your body is in a state of hyperarousal, with symptoms like tense muscles, shortness of breath, and possibly fatigue, explains Christine Celio, Ph.D., head of psychology at Calibrate, a telemedicine startup. Sound familiar? You're hardly alone. Most of us can identify with this common response to stress.

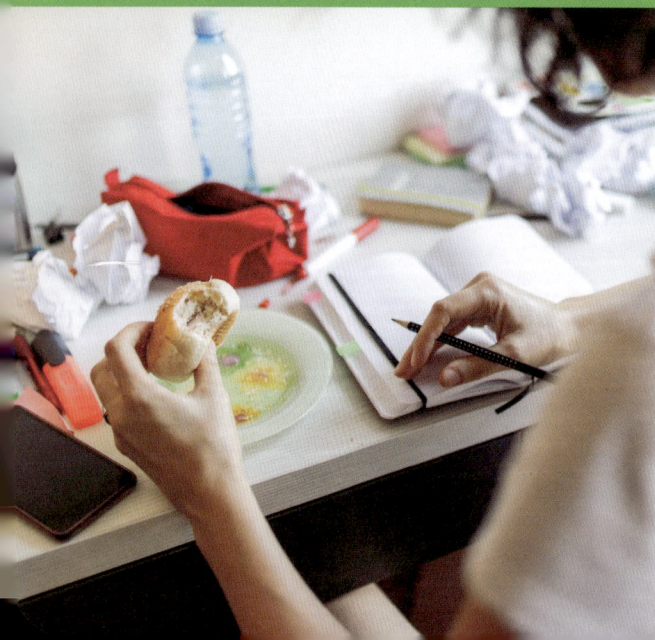

Try This Now

The first thing to do if you're concerned about your stress-eating habits is to pay attention, Celio says. When you are eating foods that don't serve your health goals, take note of whether you are truly hungry or just want to eat, and how your thoughts are impacting how much and what you're eating. "Identifying what is driving the behavior will help decide what to do next," she says. Next, write things down. "Writing down everything can clarify where the stress is coming from and can give you the perspective that while eating a bowl of pretzels does not, in fact, fix the faucet, maybe YouTubing how to do it does," Celio says.

17 Monday

18 Tuesday

19 Wednesday

20 Thursday ☽

21 Friday

22 Saturday

23 Sunday

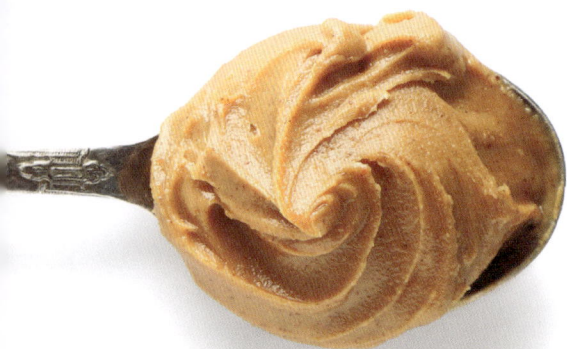

August
24–30
2026

M	T	W	T	F	S	S
					1	2
3	4	5	6	7	8	9
10	11	12	13	14	15	16
17	18	19	20	21	22	23
24	25	26	27	28	29	30
31						

MAKE MAGNESIUM A PRIORITY

Stress can cause your body to use more magnesium than usual, which can limit your body's ability to do other tasks with the nutrient, says Scott Keatley, R.D., co-owner of Keatley Medical Nutrition Therapy. "In addition, magnesium can help reduce the release of stress hormones like cortisol," he says. "It's like a natural chill pill."

Try It Now

There are a lot of foods that are high in magnesium, and Keatley recommends trying to get more of the nutrient in your diet from food first. These are the most magnesium-rich foods, according to the NIH:

Pumpkin seeds	Soymilk
Chia seeds	Black beans
Almonds	Edamame
Spinach	Peanut butter
Cashews	Potato with skin
Peanuts	Brown rice
Shredded wheat	Plain yogurt

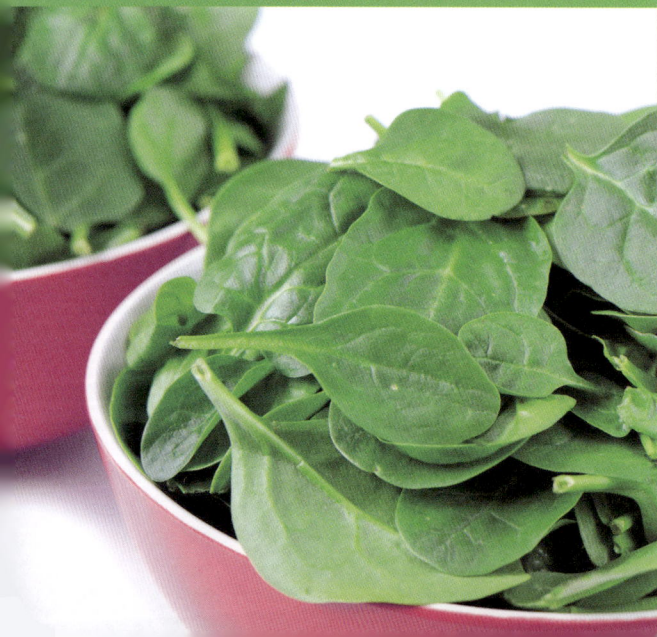

24 Monday ○

25 Tuesday

26 Wednesday

27 Thursday

28 Friday ○

29 Saturday

30 Sunday

SEPTEMBER 2026

MONDAY	TUESDAY	WEDNESDAY	THURSDAY
	1	2	3
7 Labor Day	8	9	10
14	15	16	17
21	22 First Day of Fall	23	24
28	29	30	

FRIDAY	SATURDAY	SUNDAY
4 ◑	5	6
11 Rosh Hashanah Begins ●	12	13
18 ◐	19	20 Yom Kippur Begins
25	26 ○	27

EAT WELL

Swap Out Sweetened Drinks. Per new research, downing two liters or more of sugar-sweetened or artificially sweetened beverages per week is associated with increased risk of atrial fibrillation (irregular heartbeat). Jazz up plain or sparkling H_2O or unsweetened iced tea with fruit, herbs, or botanicals.

AUGUST

M	T	W	T	F	S	S
					1	2
3	4	5	6	7	8	9
10	11	12	13	14	15	16
17	18	19	20	21	22	23
24	25	26	27	28	29	30
31						

OCTOBER

M	T	W	T	F	S	S
			1	2	3	4
5	6	7	8	9	10	11
12	13	14	15	16	17	18
19	20	21	22	23	24	25
26	27	28	29	30	31	

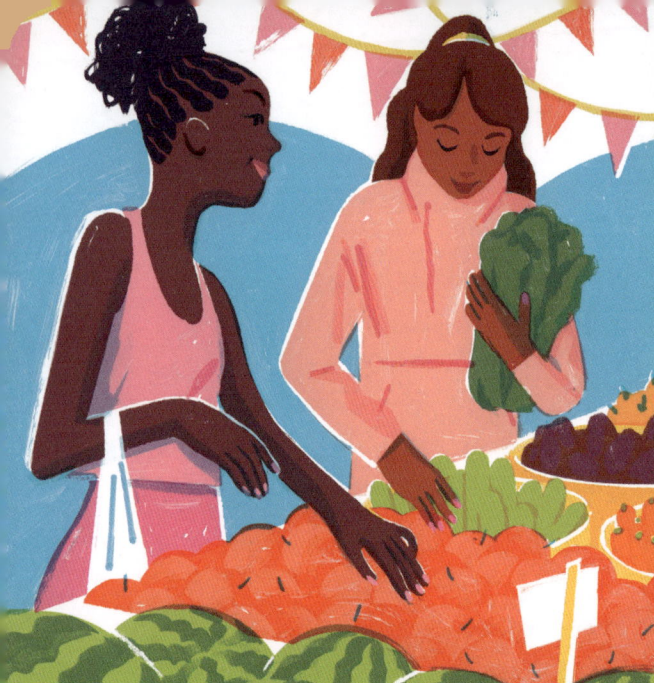

August 31– September 6

2026

M	T	W	T	F	S	S
31	1	2	3	4	5	6
7	8	9	10	11	12	13
14	15	16	17	18	19	20
21	22	23	24	25	26	27
28	29	30				

VISIT A FARMERS' MARKET

Heads up, outdoor market fans! Summertime means local farmstands are piled high with fruits and veggies right now. Seasonal produce is at peak flavor and nutrition, so now is the time to enjoy your faves at their prime, says nutrition consultant Jaclyn London, R.D., a podcast host and the author of *Dressing on the Side (and Other Diet Myths Debunked)*.

Why It Works

"Eating locally allows you to explore the nuances in taste and nutritional density that are unique to your location. Plus, there's so much joy in discovering what's new and fresh each week—and it's a great activity to do while traveling too," London says. Next time you're browsing, chat up farmers or whoever is working behind the various stands. "They love sharing their knowledge of what's tasting great, explaining unfamiliar items, and offering tips for using what you choose," London says. Knowing exactly where your food comes from—and who grew it—can bring you a sense of connectedness and calm to your next meal.

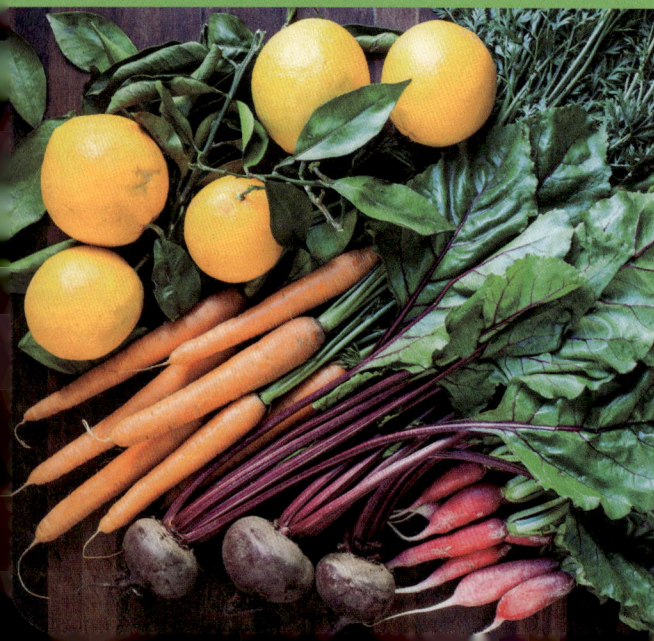

31 Monday

1 Tuesday

2 Wednesday

3 Thursday

4 Friday ◐

5 Saturday

6 Sunday

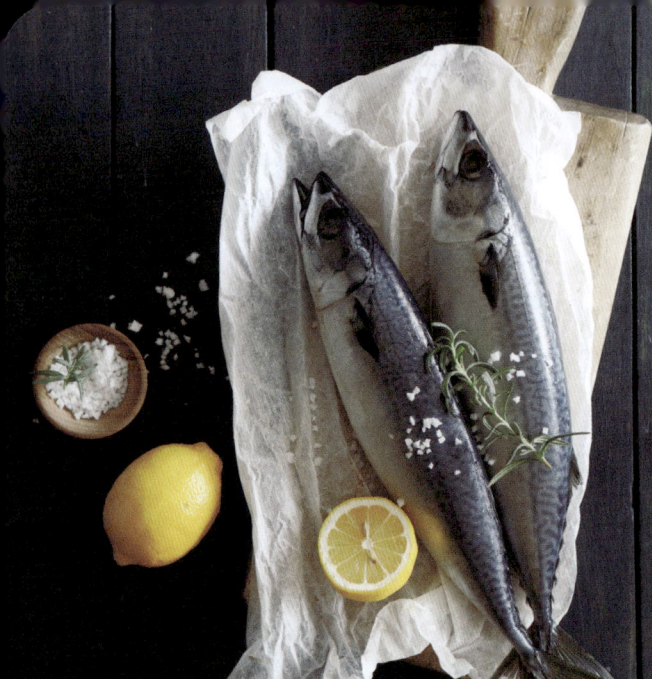

September
7–13
2026

M	T	W	T	F	S	S
	1	2	3	4	5	6
7	8	9	10	11	12	13
14	15	16	17	18	19	20
21	22	23	24	25	26	27
28	29	30				

BOOST YOUR OMEGA-3s

Today, figure out a delicious way to get more of these nutritional powerhouses into your life. Omega-3 consumption may slow cognitive decline, lessen anxiety and brain fog, and improve mood. Research suggests that omega-3s reduce inflammation in the gut-brain axis and can also improve cardiovascular health. So what are you waiting for?

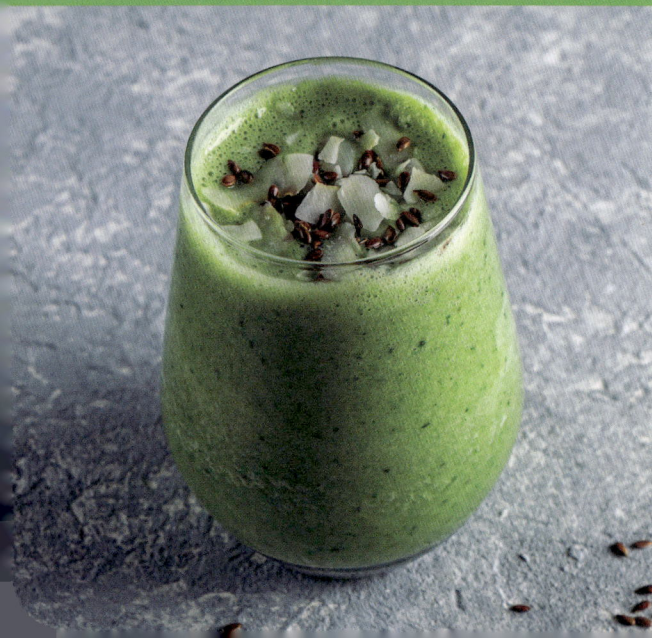

Try It Now

Fatty fish such as salmon, mackerel, and herring are one way to get your omega-3s, but if you are vegan—or just don't like fish—you can still get a powerful boost from plant-based foods such as walnuts and flaxseeds. (Use them in a smoothie, sprinkle them on yogurt, or mix them into a salad.) If none of those options appeal to you, ask your doctor if you should take a supplement, then look for one with 1,000 mg of fish oil, including EPA and DHA.

7 Monday Labor Day

8 Tuesday

9 Wednesday

10 Thursday

11 Friday ● Rosh Hashanah Begins

12 Saturday

13 Sunday

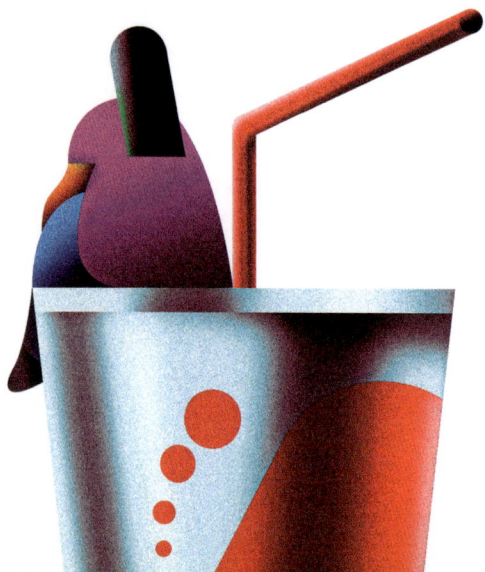

September 14–20

2026

M	T	W	T	F	S	S
	1	2	3	4	5	6
7	8	9	10	11	12	13
14	**15**	**16**	**17**	**18**	**19**	**20**
21	22	23	24	25	26	27
28	29	30				

DEEP-CLEAN YOUR DIET

There's a well-studied connection between the gut and the brain, says Uma Naidoo, M.D., director of nutritional and metabolic psychiatry at Massachusetts General Hospital and the author of *Calm Your Mind with Food*. So consider replacing brain-sapping foods with delicious alternatives that can reduce the inflammation tied to mood disorders.

Here's What to Do

Foods closely tied to inflammation tend to be prominent in the standard American diet, including highly refined ultraprocessed foods, fried foods, fast foods, refined carbohydrates, and sugary drinks. Dr. Naidoo recommends these strategies:

- Clear out sugary canned or bottled drinks and restock with herbal teas.
- Swap out processed snacks for brain-healthy hummus, nut butter, and extra-dark natural chocolate.
- Try to focus on a plant-forward diet while including a clean protein of your choice, such as tofu or chicken, with each meal.

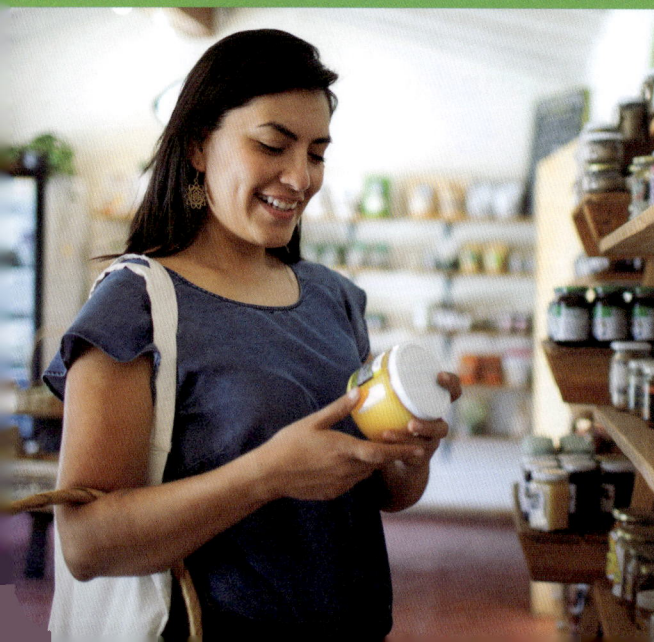

14 Monday

15 Tuesday

16 Wednesday

17 Thursday

18 Friday ◑

19 Saturday

20 Sunday Yom Kippur Begins

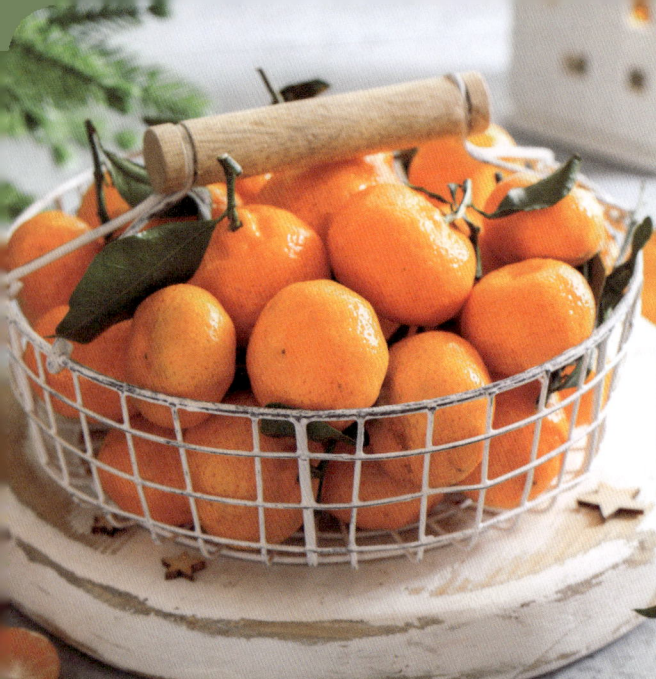

September 21–27

2026

M	T	W	T	F	S	S
	1	2	3	4	5	6
7	8	9	10	11	12	13
14	15	16	17	18	19	20
21	**22**	**23**	**24**	**25**	**26**	**27**
28	29	30				

PEEL A CLEMENTINE

The simple act of peeling a clementine is a mindful relaxation technique. "Peeling citrus fruit is a mini-meditative moment—you have to drop whatever you're doing to engage both hands," says Susan Albers, a psychologist at the Cleveland Clinic and the author of *Eating Mindfully*, a *New York Times* bestseller.

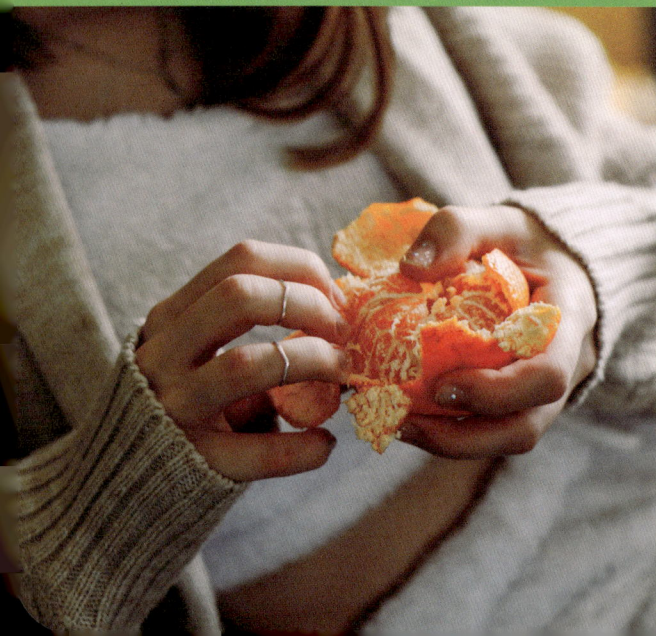

Why It Works

Even the smell of citrus has been shown to promote calm—which might just quell your urge to binge on a less nutritious option. For optimum relaxation, slowly peel the fruit in a spiral pattern as you breathe in deeply to inhale the scent. When you're done peeling, eat the fruit one segment at a time, taking a moment to savor each bite.

Some research suggests that when you're feeling stressed out, eating healthier foods can help restore your mood just as well as the traditional comfort foods that are so easy to turn to.

21 Monday

22 Tuesday First Day of Fall

23 Wednesday

24 Thursday

25 Friday

26 Saturday ○

27 Sunday

FALL
AGE-PROOF
YOUR BODY

It might sound like science fiction if it weren't so ordinary: Our bones break and mend...we burn a hand and it heals...we forget words and remember in a flash. The body has an astounding ability to bounce back that can feel like a miracle of sorts.

However, it can be stressful to realize how much our innate healing power naturally slows down as we grow older. We lose a few more words, or more days elapse between a scrape and smooth skin. Resources for repair take longer to marshal their forces.

But we can help our body retain resiliency—that incredible ability to absorb stress, strain, and pain and then adapt and recover. Physicians and researchers are making fascinating discoveries about how we can build a more resilient system at any age. Here's exactly what you can do to stay calm about the aging process and keep your body bouncing back.

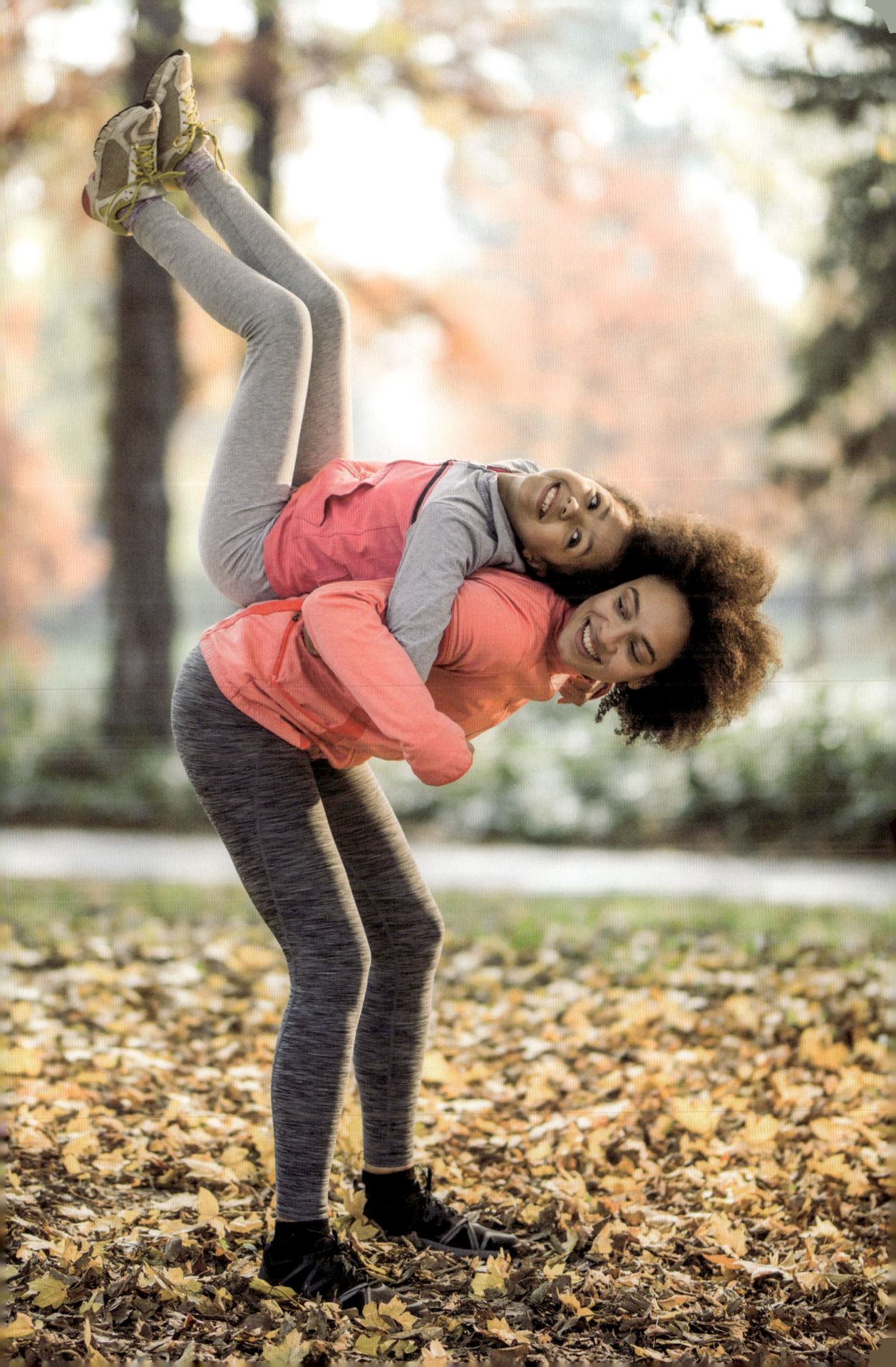

A Stress-Free Guide to Whole-Body Health

We may not yet be able to online-order a personalized fountain of youth, but science is revealing important ways we can improve our innate healing abilities that aren't just science fiction. Here's a rundown of how you can tap into your inner resources and claim the power of your own resilience!

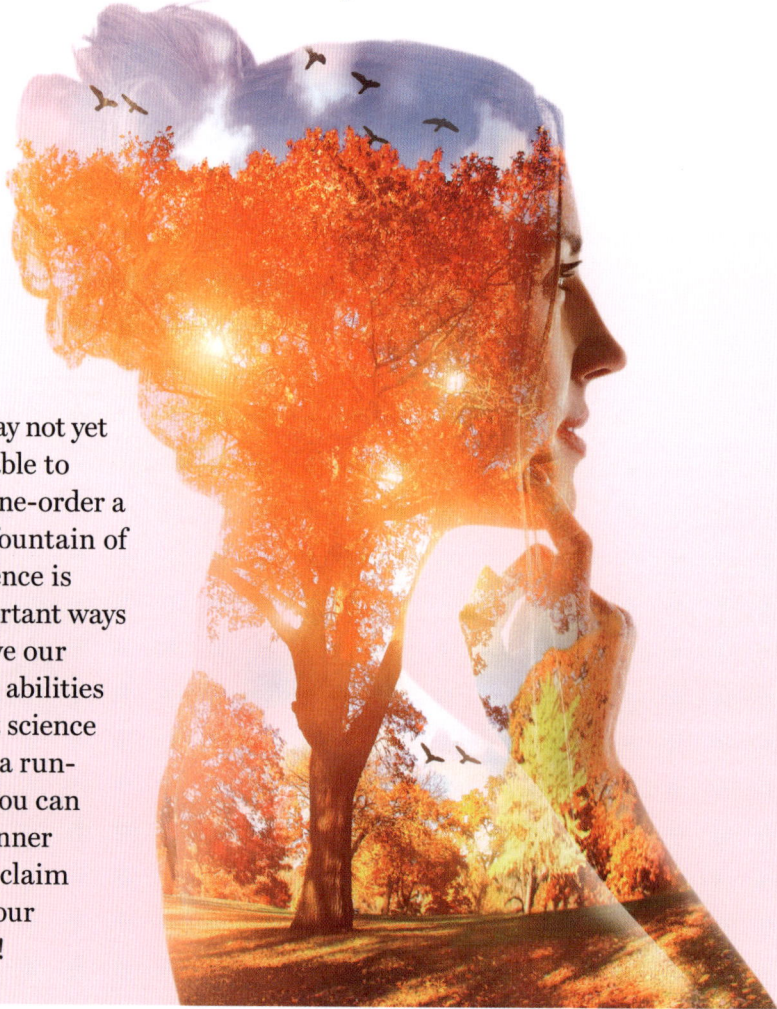

Brain

OUR BRAIN tends to shrink as we age, explains Richard Hunter, Ph.D., director of the Lab of Neuroepigenetics and Genomics at the University of Massachusetts Boston. Certain cognitive abilities can suffer: For instance, after age 60 our perceptual speed declines and we need more time to notice a shift in the environment, like a traffic light change. Our verbal and spatial memory can suffer too, making it harder to remember names and where we've left things. Sound at all familiar?

While this is a normal aspect of aging, you can fight it. "Brain resilience generally means holding on to more brain volume and cognitive function longer," Hunter says. He knows scientists he describes as "supersharp" who have devoted their lives to learning and are cognitively intact well into their 80s.

These may be what the National Institutes of Health deems "cognitive super-agers," who perform like people 20 years younger on memory tests. Want to be one of them? For a more resilient brain, consider the following:

Socialize smarter. To build tomorrow's cognitive reserve, Hunter suggests increasing your social and intellectual engagement. That could mean meeting new people and enjoying new experiences, such as having a chat at the bus stop en route to a new destination. Participation in regular social activities and tasks—calling your cousin or catching up with a coworker—can help too.

"Humans are social animals, and our connections have helped us succeed as a species," Hunter says. "In a sense we need to socialize to survive, so building good social connections seems to protect you from aging's worst effects."

In one study of people 65 and older, loneliness was connected with accelerated cognitive decline even after accounting for factors including depression and health conditions.

Find activities that combine interpersonal components with educational or exercise ones, such as participating in a trail cleanup, rock climbing in a gym with a friend, singing in a choir, or playing cards. Taking partner-style dance lessons gives you triple benefits— learning, moving, and socializing.

Skin

A SKINNED KNEE took a week or so to heal when you were a child. If it now seems to take twice as long (or longer), you're not imagining it. As we age, cells in our three skin layers don't turn over the way they used to—a necessary process for clearing out damage and making repairs. Cell turnover slows down even more quickly if we have failed to wear sunscreen (oops), smoked, or been exposed to air pollution.

By our mid-40s, our skin tears more easily and forms wrinkles. "If we don't invest in fixing the machinery that turns over the skin, it goes to sleep," says Abigail Waldman, M.D., clinical director of the Mohs and Dermatologic Surgery Center at Brigham and Women's Hospital and an assistant professor at Harvard Medical School. Here's how to wake your skin up again.

STRESS IT OUT. The primary method for restoring skin's natural resilience is to injure it. Hear us out: Two approaches— using retinoids and processes like microneedling—boost resilience by stressing

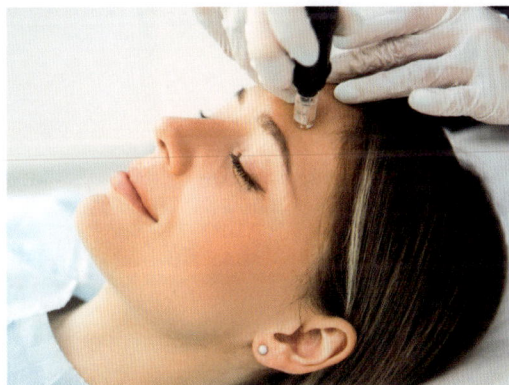

skin and instigating cell turnover. Retinoids, typically used in facial creams, essentially reawaken your cell turnover machinery, which can then strengthen the skin's protective function, limit moisture loss, and protect collagen. That can result in smoother, clearer skin that can bounce back from an injury more quickly. Plus, the ingredient will refresh hands, knees, and feet, Dr. Waldman says. Products with higher percentages of retinoids will revive the skin's machinery faster, but the lower percentages (such as 1%) found in over-the-counter formulas will work too—you just might need to wait a year or so to see noticeable results.

That's OK, Dr. Waldman says, if you view it as part of a rest-of-your-life routine, not a fix-it-fast process. Meanwhile, procedures like chemical peels, microneedling, and microdermabrasion lead to nanoinjuries in the outer layers of the skin, creating more collagen and elastin. It's like exercise, Dr. Waldman says: "To build muscle strength, you're creating tiny injuries your body will fix and make stronger." A skincare specialist can help you find the right treatment and number of sessions.

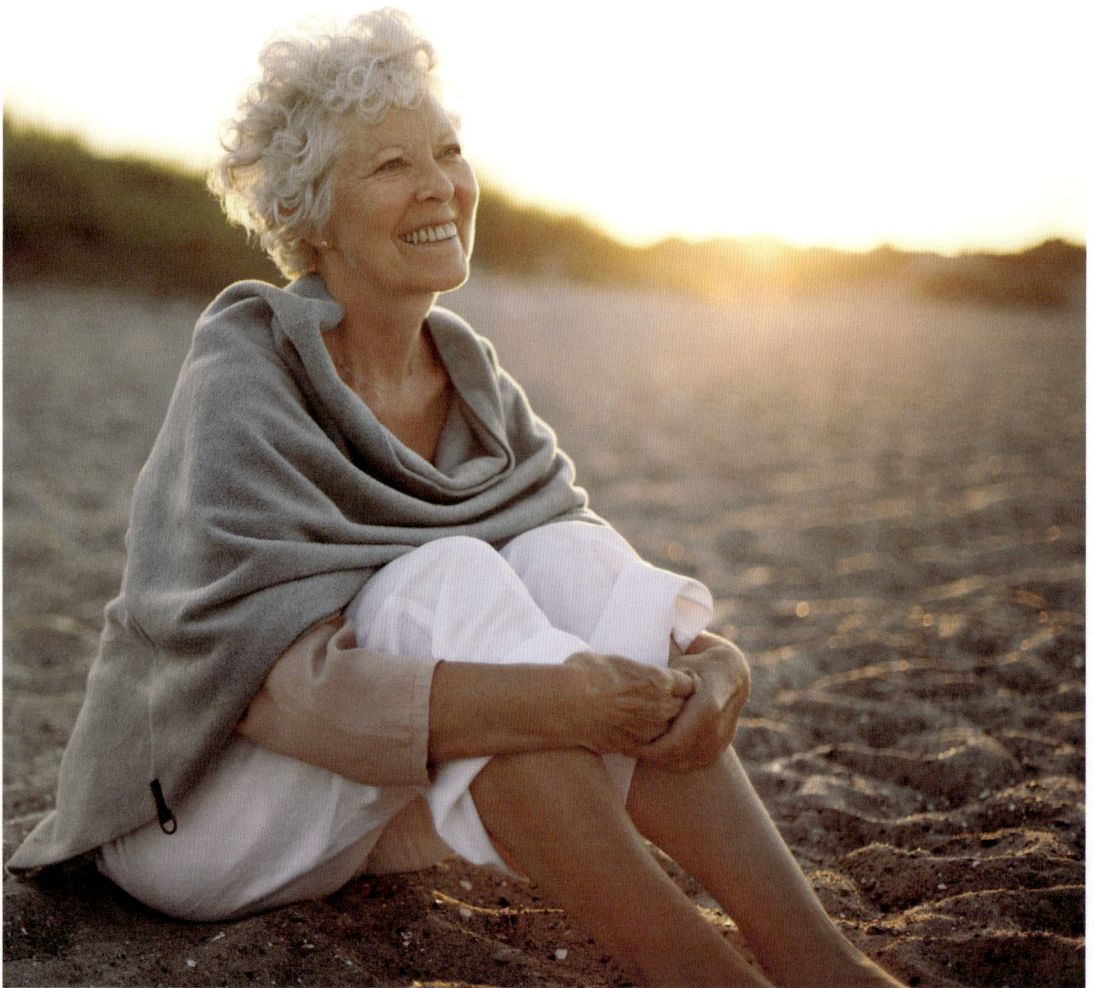

Bones, Muscles and Joints

WHETHER YOU'RE WALKING, cooking, or trying a TikTok dance, your bones, muscles, joints, and cartilage move your body as an integrated system. But this system starts to fall apart in our third and fourth decades, says Marco Brotto, Ph.D., MPharm, director of the Bone-Muscle Research Center at the University of Texas at Arlington. Bones break more easily because of calcium loss, while muscles lose mass and strength because of age-related loss called sarcopenia.

By age 35 to 40, 1% to 2% of muscle mass is lost yearly, with more rapid deterioration after age 65 for women and 70 for men. Because of a negative feedback loop, feeble muscles lead to frailer joints, cartilage tears, and weaker bones. As a result, 30% of adults over 65 have trouble with everyday movement such as walking. To reverse course and build more resilience, take action now, Brotto says. Doing so can help you maintain mobility and improve your coordination and strength so you will be less likely to endure a sprain, fracture, or break—and if you do, you'll recover more quickly. Here's how to build a more resilient musculoskeletal system:

STRETCH AND STRENGTH-TRAIN. Try body-weight moves or a whole-body resistance band workout. Not sure where to start? Begin with squats, says Brotto. "Squats are among the most wonderful exercises because they engage the largest muscles in the body," he says. Aim to get 15 minutes of strength training every day or 30 minutes every other day.

In addition, you can increase flexibility, range, and balance through daily stretching and balance work if possible—whether you do yoga, Pilates, tai chi, or simple stretching. "The most effective intervention for prevention of falls of all tested to date is tai chi," Brotto says. You can also increase joint mobility through stretching, which limbers up the soft tissues (tendon, muscle, skin, fat, and fascia) connecting and surrounding bone and internal organs. "The most important thing is to stay as active as possible for as long as you can. Do not underestimate the power of your own body, and make sure to reach out to a friend or consider joining a gym or a club or doing volunteering that will require you to stay active. Aim to live longer, but also stronger," he says.

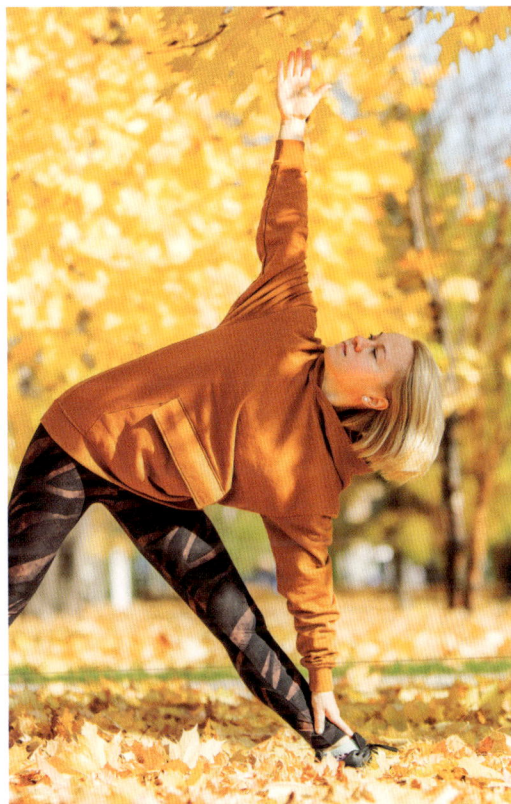

OCTOBER 2026

MONDAY	TUESDAY	WEDNESDAY	THURSDAY
			1
5	6	7	8
12 Indigenous Peoples' Day	13	14	15
19	20	21	22
26 ○	27	28	29

FRIDAY	SATURDAY	SUNDAY
2	3 ◑	4
9	10 ●	11
16	17	18 ◐
23	24	25
30	31 Halloween	

SEPTEMBER

M	T	W	T	F	S	S
	1	2	3	4	5	6
7	8	9	10	11	12	13
14	15	16	17	18	19	20
21	22	23	24	25	26	27
28	29	30				

NOVEMBER

M	T	W	T	F	S	S
						1
2	3	4	5	6	7	8
9	10	11	12	13	14	15
16	17	18	19	20	21	22
23	24	25	26	27	28	29
30						

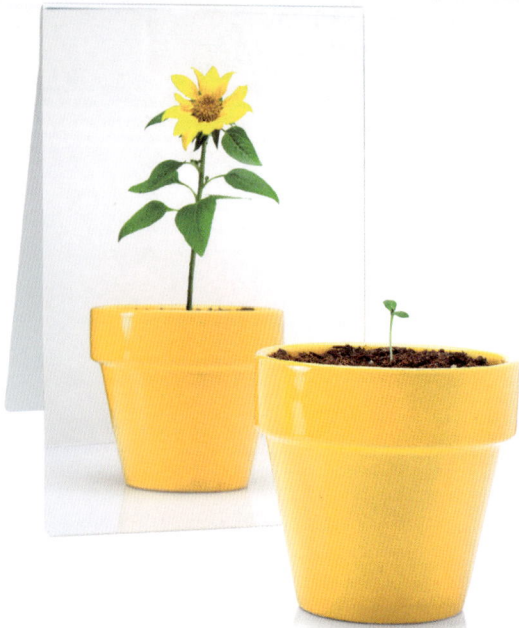

September 28 – October 4

2026

M	T	W	T	F	S	S
28	29	30	1	2	3	4
5	6	7	8	9	10	11
12	13	14	15	16	17	18
19	20	21	22	23	24	25
26	27	28	29	30	31	

STAY HOPEFUL

Researchers in Finland published a fascinating study in which they found that very cynical older people had higher rates of dementia. Why? Negative stress could be the culprit; we know, for instance, that high levels of cortisol, the stress hormone, can have a very unhealthy effect on the brain and may stop people from thinking clearly.

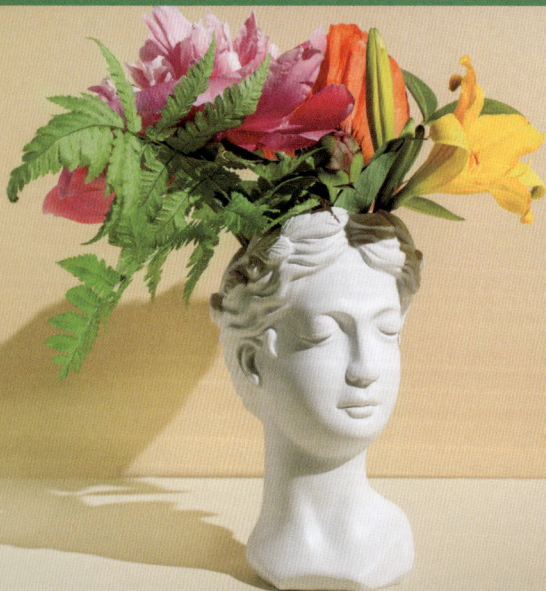

What to Do

"A positive attitude may be associated with good cognitive aging," says Neill Graff-Radford, M.D., a professor of neurology at the Mayo Clinic in Jacksonville, FL. "I have met a number of centenarians, including Holocaust survivors, and they light up the room when they enter it."

If your worldview tends to be cynical (defined as a belief that others are generally selfish or dishonest), start to notice when that attitude comes up and, in those moments, try to actively change your mindset.

28 Monday

29 Tuesday

30 Wednesday

1 Thursday

2 Friday

3 Saturday ◑

4 Sunday

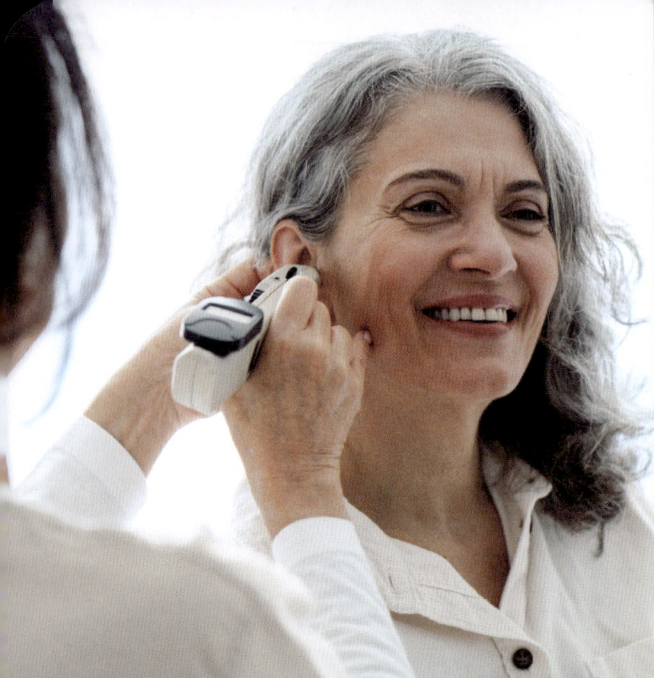

October
5–11
2026

M	T	W	T	F	S	S
			1	2	3	4
5	6	7	8	9	10	11
12	13	14	15	16	17	18
19	20	21	22	23	24	25
26	27	28	29	30	31	

SCHEDULE A HEARING TEST

Do you feel like people are mumbling more? Are you hitting the TV volume button harder? Don't stress out—get your hearing tested instead. Research at Johns Hopkins found that even mild hearing loss doubled the risk for dementia, and moderate loss tripled it. Plus, straining to hear makes your brain work harder, which can affect memory and thinking.

What We Know

There are a couple of reasons why not being able to see and hear well could contribute to dementia, in particular. Stimulation from all our senses helps keep the brain's functions buzzing along. When that stimulation is impaired, neurons start to die off. And there's a behavioral factor as well: Embarrassment about losing one's hearing can make a person start to socially isolate— another dementia risk factor. And should you find yourself in need of a hearing aid, don't stress about it. Multiple studies have confirmed that people who use them have lower rates of depression, anxiety, and loneliness.

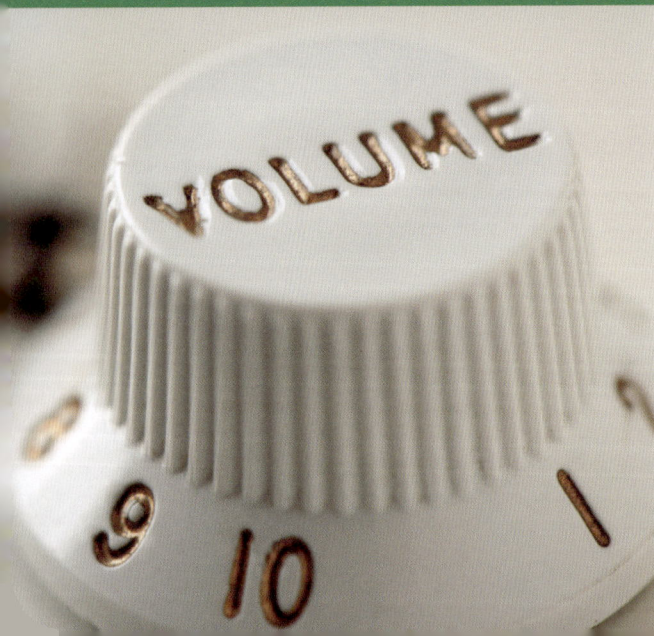

5 Monday ○

6 Tuesday

7 Wednesday

8 Thursday

9 Friday

10 Saturday ●

11 Sunday

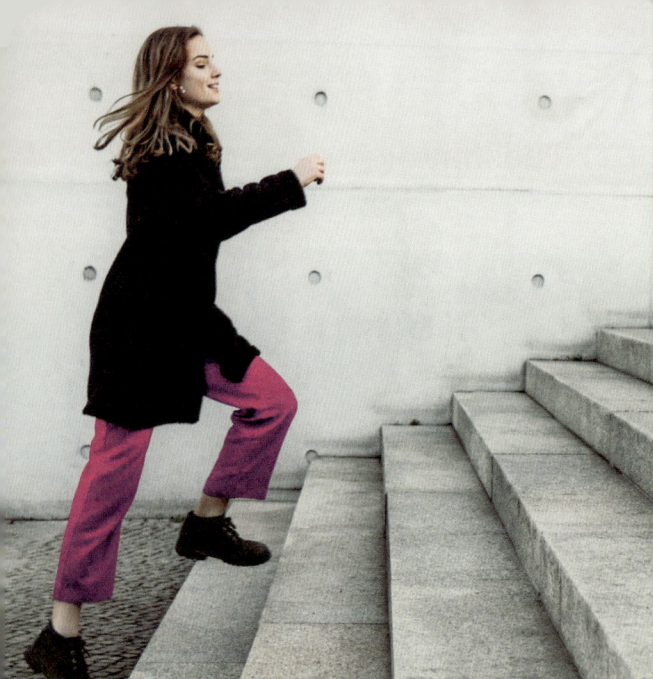

October
12–18
2026

M	T	W	T	F	S	S
			1	2	3	4
5	6	7	8	9	10	11
12	13	14	15	16	17	18
19	20	21	22	23	24	25
26	27	28	29	30	31	

TAKE THE STAIRS

For every flight of stairs you climb every day, your brain age drops by 0.58 year, according to research from Concordia University. Even better is when you learn to like that upward hike. "Do the exercise you enjoy doing," says Thomas R. Vidic, M.D., a fellow of the American Academy of Neurology who practices at the Elkhart Clinic in Elkhart, IN.

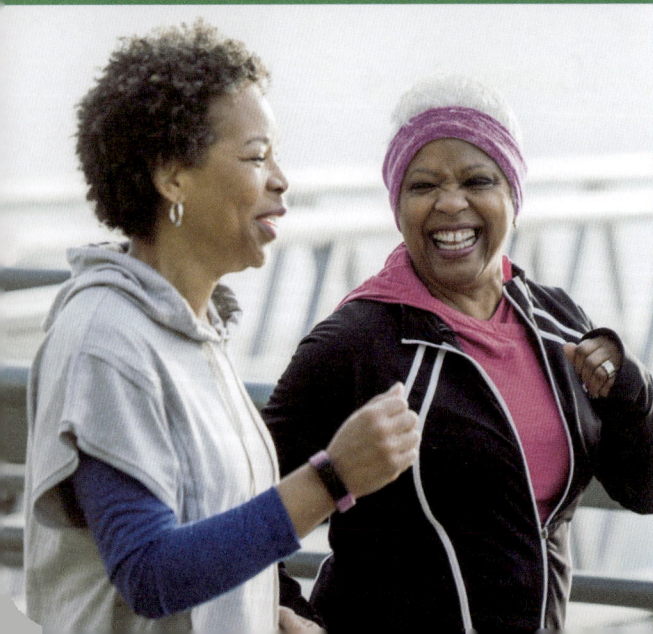

Try It Now

Focusing on activities you enjoy enables your brain to release hormones that will help you stick to your workout. So put on your headphones, cue up a playlist you love, and carve out time to climb stairs or get similar exercise at work or home for a total of 150 minutes per week. Other strategies to try? Sign up for that salsa dancing class you've been curious about, or enlist a couple of neighbors to create a weekly walking group. You'll get the double benefit of exercise and social connection.

12 Monday Indigenous Peoples' Day

13 Tuesday

14 Wednesday

15 Thursday

16 Friday

17 Saturday

18 Sunday ◑

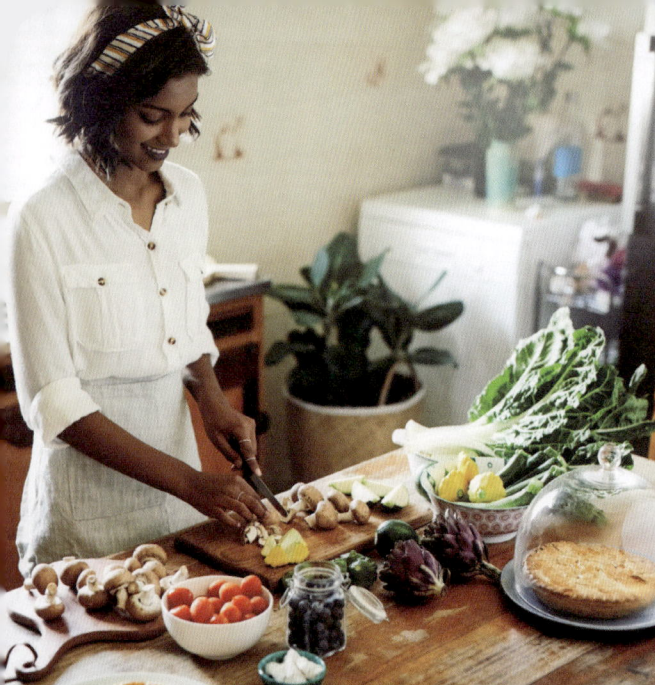

October
19–25
2026

M	T	W	T	F	S	S
			1	2	3	4
5	6	7	8	9	10	11
12	13	14	15	16	17	18
19	20	21	22	23	24	25
26	27	28	29	30	31	

TRY THE MIND DIET

What exactly are we talking about? The MIND Diet (Mediterranean-DASH Intervention for Neurodegenerative Delay) is a food plan rich in leafy greens, berries, nuts, fish, and olive oil, and it even includes a little wine. Of course there are some foods to limit or avoid, too, such as red meat, butter and margarine, cheese, and fried foods.

Why It Works

Not only are MIND foods delicious, but the plan can turn back cognitive age by up to seven and a half years, according to a 2015 study. More than 900 men and women with an average age of 81.4 detailed their diets and had their cognitive function checked over a period of more than four years. In another 2015 study, participants who carefully followed the MIND diet—limiting foods like red meat, sugary treats, and fried foods—cut their Alzheimer's disease risk by 53%, and those who followed the diet pretty well cut their risk by 35%.

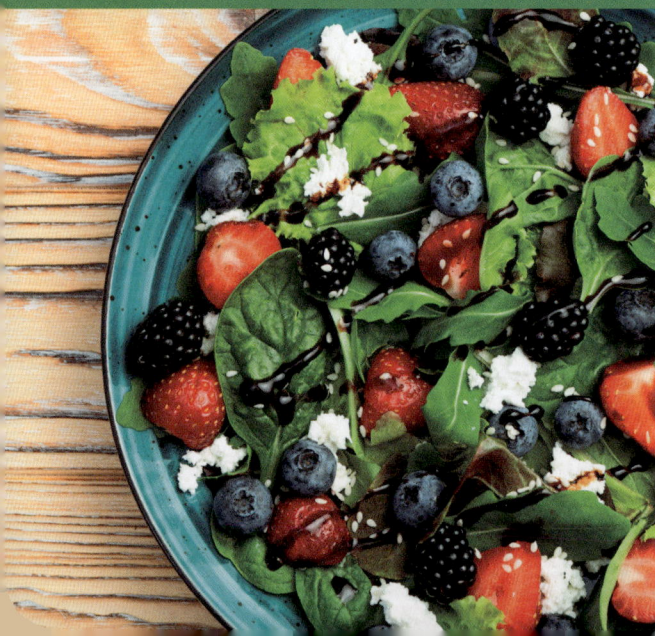

19 Monday

20 Tuesday

21 Wednesday

22 Thursday

23 Friday

24 Saturday

25 Sunday

NOVEMBER 2026

MONDAY	TUESDAY	WEDNESDAY	THURSDAY
2	3 Election Day	4	5
9 ●	10	11 Veterans Day	12
16	17 ◑	18	19
23	24 ○	25	26 Thanksgiving
30			

FRIDAY	SATURDAY	SUNDAY
		1 All Saints' Day Daylight Saving Time Ends ◑
6	**7**	**8** Diwali Begins
13	**14**	**15**
20	**21**	**22**
27	**28**	**29** First Day of Advent

AGE WELL

Love Your Years.
People with positive attitudes toward getting older tend to live longer and have fewer health issues than those who approach aging with a negative mindset, per a large body of research by Harvard's T.H. Chan School of Public Health. Positive individuals also showed better cognitive functioning and were more likely to keep up with good-for-you lifestyle habits like exercising regularly and getting quality sleep.

OCTOBER

M	T	W	T	F	S	S
			1	2	3	4
5	6	7	8	9	10	11
12	13	14	15	16	17	18
19	20	21	22	23	24	25
26	27	28	29	30	31	

DECEMBER

M	T	W	T	F	S	S
	1	2	3	4	5	6
7	8	9	10	11	12	13
14	15	16	17	18	19	20
21	22	23	24	25	26	27
28	29	30	31			

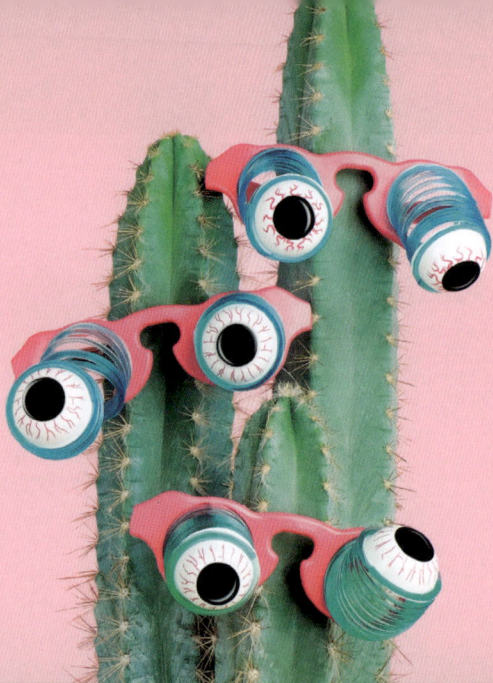

October 26–November 1

2026

M	T	W	T	F	S	S
26	27	28	29	30	31	1
2	3	4	5	6	7	8
9	10	11	12	13	14	15
16	17	18	19	20	21	22
23	24	25	26	27	28	29
30						

EASE EYESTRAIN

Your eyes get an almost constant workout from the moment they open in the morning until they close at night, so it's no wonder they feel fatigued throughout the day. "Common signs of eyestrain include redness, itching, burning, dry eye, intermittent blurring, and headaches," says Viola Kanevsky, O.D., an optometrist at Acuity NYC in Manhattan.

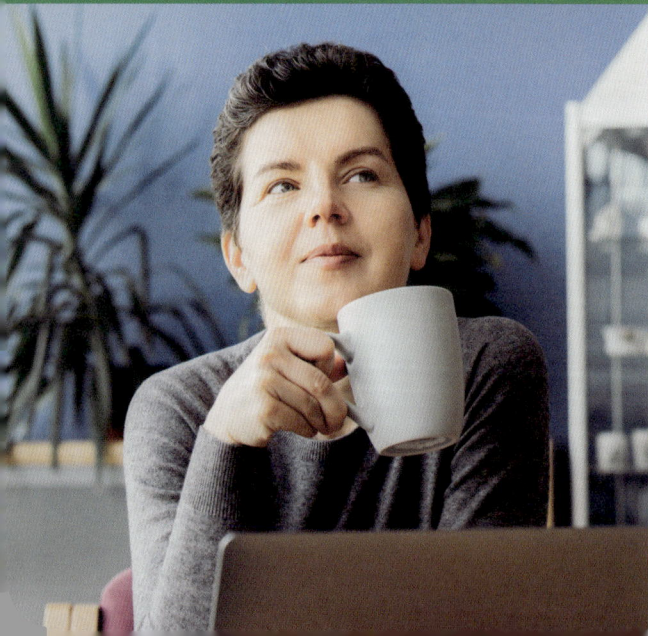

What to Do

Take frequent breaks, especially if you are on your laptop all day. Eye health experts say to follow the 20-20-20 rule: Every 20 minutes, take a 20-second (or longer) break and look at something 20 feet away. This gives your peepers a chance to rest and refocus so you can minimize eyestrain symptoms like headache and dry eye. And schedule an eye exam. If you don't already see an optometrist, seek one out; these specialists can help figure out whether your eyestrain is caused by a vision problem such as an astigmatism or presbyopia (loss of the ability to focus on nearby objects).

26 Monday ○

27 Tuesday

28 Wednesday

29 Thursday

30 Friday

31 Saturday Halloween

1 Sunday ◑ All Saints' Day
Daylight Saving Time Ends

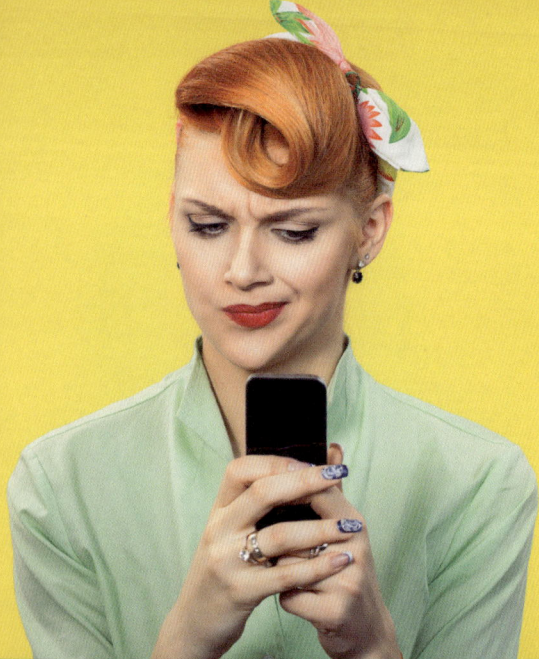

November
2–8
2026

M	T	W	T	F	S	S
						1
2	3	4	5	6	7	8
9	10	11	12	13	14	15
16	17	18	19	20	21	22
23	24	25	26	27	28	29
30						

KNOW WHEN TO LET GO

It's natural for friendships to evolve as our life stages change. In fact, one study found that while the size of a friendship network tends to be consistent over time, the people in it change: About half of a person's friendships turn over every seven years. When you have a history with someone, it can be hard to know when it's time to move on.

What to Know

There are many indications that a friendship may be too stressful and no longer worth prioritizing, but here's a list of things to consider:

- You're always the one initiating contact;
- You feel as if your energy is sapped every time you're with them;
- You can't think of anything to talk about or feel as if you can't be yourself;
- You feel that you have to call them instead of wanting to;
- You don't want to pick up when they call you;
- You find yourself being more critical and less approving of their actions.

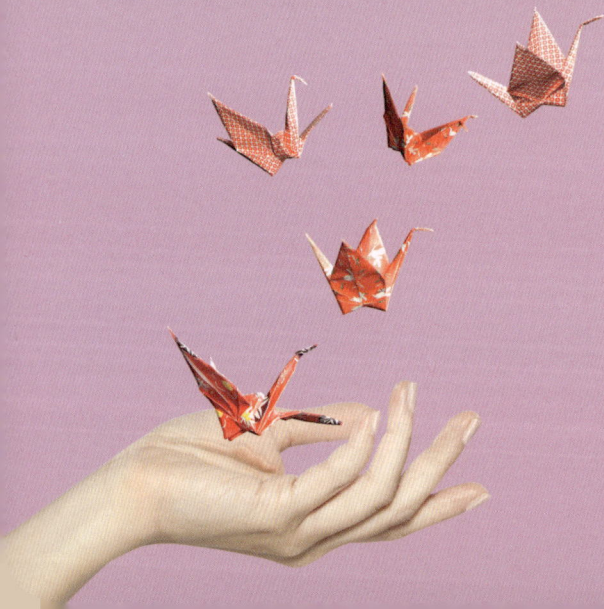

2 Monday

3 Tuesday Election Day

4 Wednesday

5 Thursday

6 Friday

7 Saturday

8 Sunday Diwali Begins

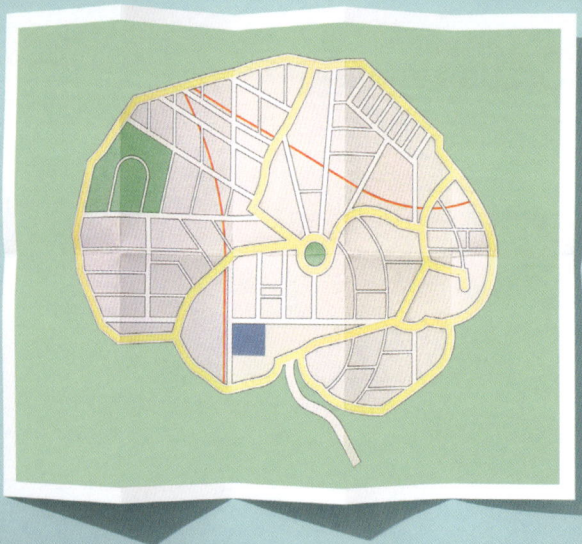

November
9–15
2026

M	T	W	T	F	S	S
						1
2	3	4	5	6	7	8
9	10	11	12	13	14	15
16	17	18	19	20	21	22
23	24	25	26	27	28	29
30						

LEARN SOMETHING NEW

Just as you build your arm muscles by exercising with increasingly heavy weights, you build new neural connections every time you challenge your brain to work harder. This helps you build a cognitive reserve, which means your brain remains adaptable even as you age, a key concept when it comes to staving off dementia.

Why It Works

Learning new things should become a habit you keep up even as your body slows down: A large study found that older adults who participated in adult education classes, played chess, or did other brain-stimulating activities had a lower risk of dementia over a 10-year period than those who did not. In fact, taking a class or learning a new skill may be one of the best things you can do to keep your brain healthy. Just make sure to choose an activity that keeps you on your toes. You want to feel like you're on the verge of being uncomfortable—you can't go on autopilot. This ensures the activity is probably working for you.

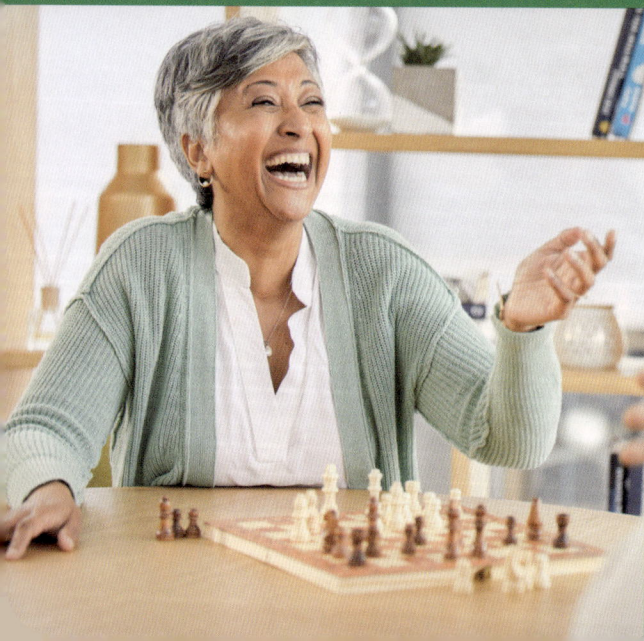

9 Monday ●

10 Tuesday

11 Wednesday Veterans Day

12 Thursday

13 Friday

14 Saturday

15 Sunday

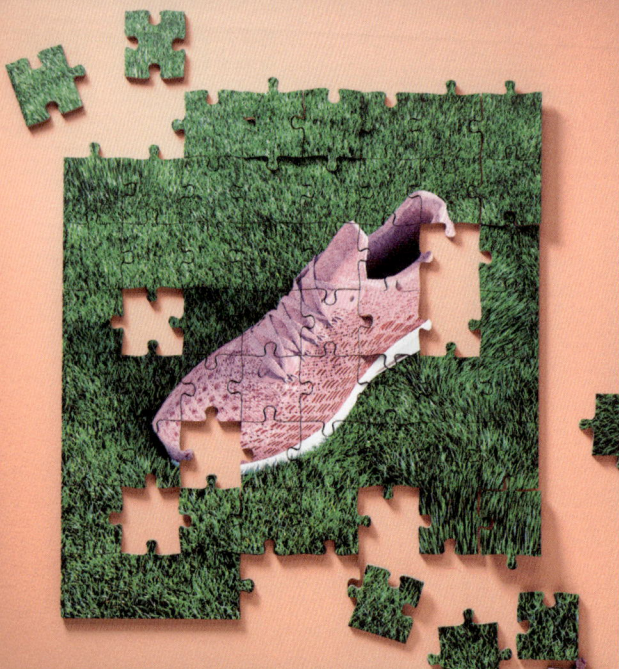

THIS WEEK
I HOPE TO . . .

November
16–22
2026

M	T	W	T	F	S	S
						1
2	3	4	5	6	7	8
9	10	11	12	13	14	15
16	17	18	19	20	21	22
23	24	25	26	27	28	29
30						

CROSS-TRAIN YOUR BRAIN

If you're on your 500th Wordle, you may want to put the phone down—at least for a bit. When it comes to the benefits of puzzles for brain function, Zaldy S. Tan, M.D., M.P.H., director of the Memory & Healthy Aging Program at Cedars-Sinai, recommends doing other brain-boosting activities, not just repeating the same types of exercises.

Try It Now

"Brain games, crossword puzzles, and Sudoku are meant to challenge specific areas of the brain, but our minds are complex, and different areas serve different functions," he says. Instead, try puzzles one day, read a book the next; take a Spanish class, go to lunch with friends. Whatever you choose, engaging in a mix of activities may strengthen brain circuits and stimulate new brain connections, which can help you function if typical brain networks are disrupted due to disease. "Think of it like cross-training for the brain, because different activities give you a better chance of having the totality of your mind stimulated and engaged," says Dr. Tan.

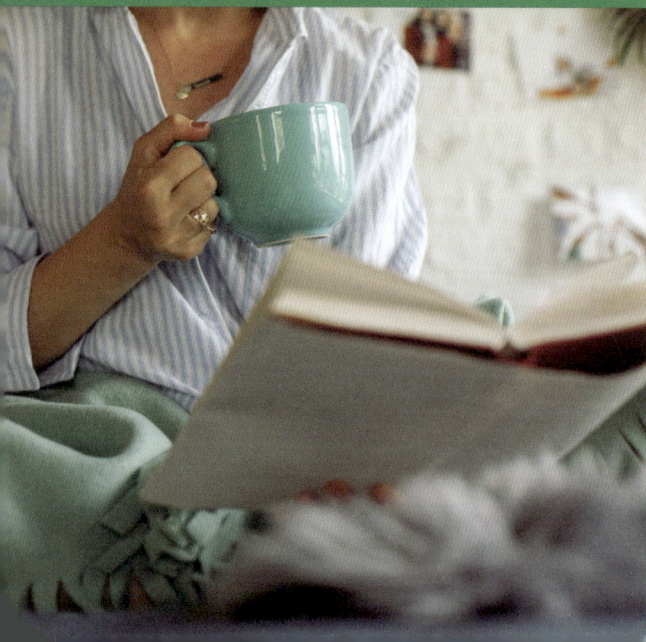

16 Monday

17 Tuesday ◑

18 Wednesday

19 Thursday

20 Friday

21 Saturday

22 Sunday

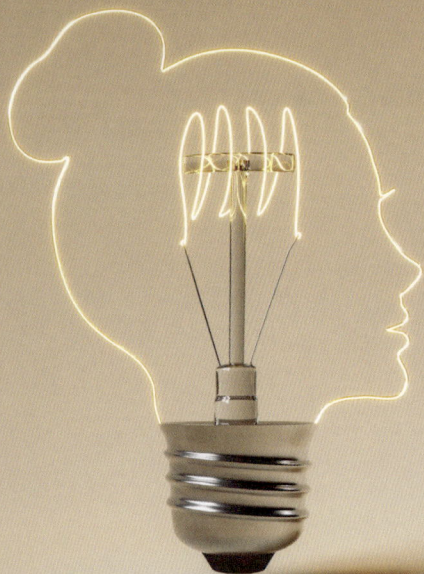

November 23–29

2026

M	T	W	T	F	S	S
						1
2	3	4	5	6	7	8
9	10	11	12	13	14	15
16	17	18	19	20	21	22
23	24	25	26	27	28	29
30						

SHARPEN YOUR MEMORY—WITH A PEN

Do you remember things better when you jot them down? There's a reason for that, says Lisa Genova, a neuroscientist and author of the bestseller *Remember: The Science of Memory and the Art of Forgetting*. Basically, the more points of attachment there are to a memory, the more possibilities you have for accessing it later.

Why It Works

"Our brains are not designed to remember to do things later," says Genova. "This is called prospective memory, and it is unreliable in everyone. People think, *Oh, it's cheating if I use a to-do list or a checklist. I should be working that part of my brain, or it's going to get weaker.* But it's actually very good practice to outsource the job to a written list. Prospective memory requires the exact right cue in the exact right place at the exact right time. Don't expect that your brain will remember anything you need to do later. It isn't cheating to write things down."

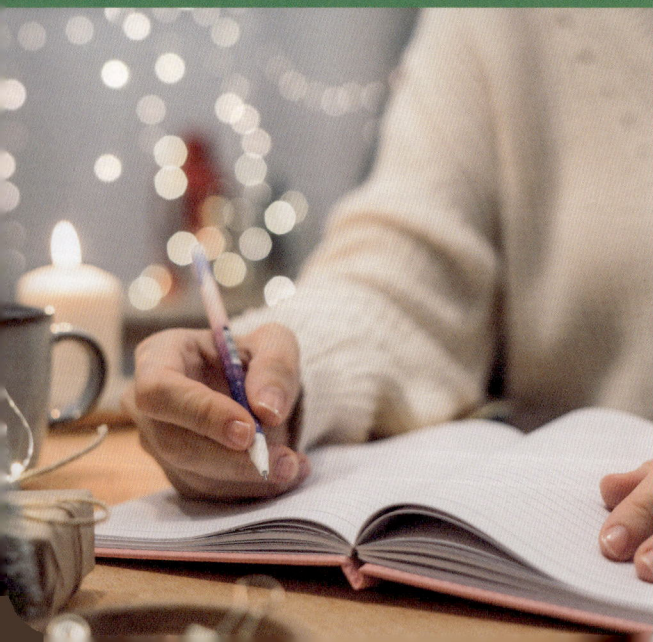

23 Monday

24 Tuesday ○

25 Wednesday

26 Thursday Thanksgiving

27 Friday ☽

28 Saturday

29 Sunday First Day of Advent

DECEMBER 2026

MONDAY	TUESDAY	WEDNESDAY	THURSDAY
	1 ◑	2	3
7	8	9 ●	10
14	15	16	17 ◐
21 First Day of Winter	22	23	24 Christmas Eve ○
28	29	30 ◑	31 New Year's Eve

FRIDAY	SATURDAY	SUNDAY
4 Hanukkah Begins	**5**	**6**
11	**12**	**13**
18	**19**	**20**
25 Christmas Day	**26** Kwanzaa Begins	**27**

AGE WELL

Give Thanks. Being grateful is good for you. Research shows that appreciating blessings both big (say, a promotion at work) and small (like spotting a pretty bird in the park) can boost happiness, and people who regularly practice gratitude tend to sleep better and have a lower risk of depression and anxiety. What better time than the holiday season to start or nurture a gratitude ritual?

NOVEMBER

M	T	W	T	F	S	S
						1
2	3	4	5	6	7	8
9	10	11	12	13	14	15
16	17	18	19	20	21	22
23	24	25	26	27	28	29
30						

JANUARY

M	T	W	T	F	S	S
				1	2	3
4	5	6	7	8	9	10
11	12	13	14	15	16	17
18	19	20	21	22	23	24
25	26	27	28	29	30	31

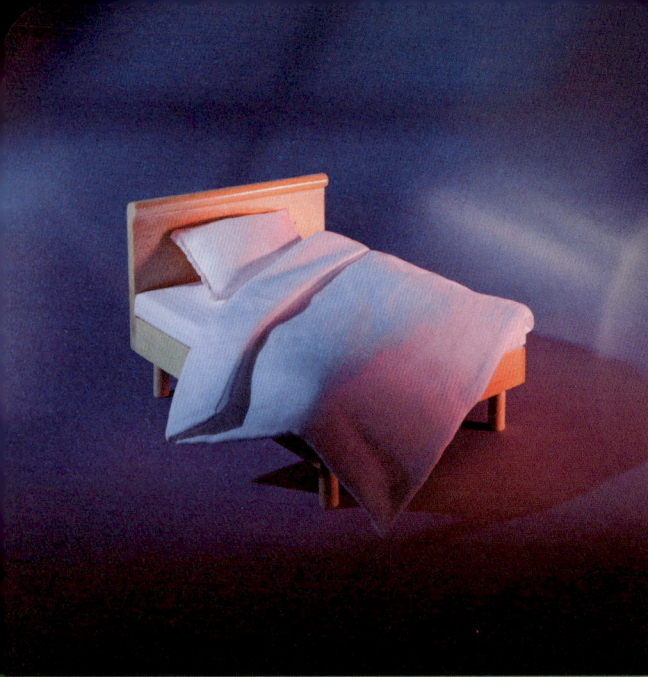

November 30–
December 6
2026

M	T	W	T	F	S	S
30	1	2	3	4	5	6
7	8	9	10	11	12	13
14	15	16	17	18	19	20
21	22	23	24	25	26	27
28	29	30	31			

STRATEGIZE FOR BETTER SLEEP

Chronic lack of sleep can be stressful, especially when it comes to your blood pressure and risk of heart disease. When we snooze, our blood pressure drops to its lowest point of the day, which helps us maintain healthy blood pressure during our waking hours, says Rebecca Robbins, Ph.D., a sleep expert for Oura.

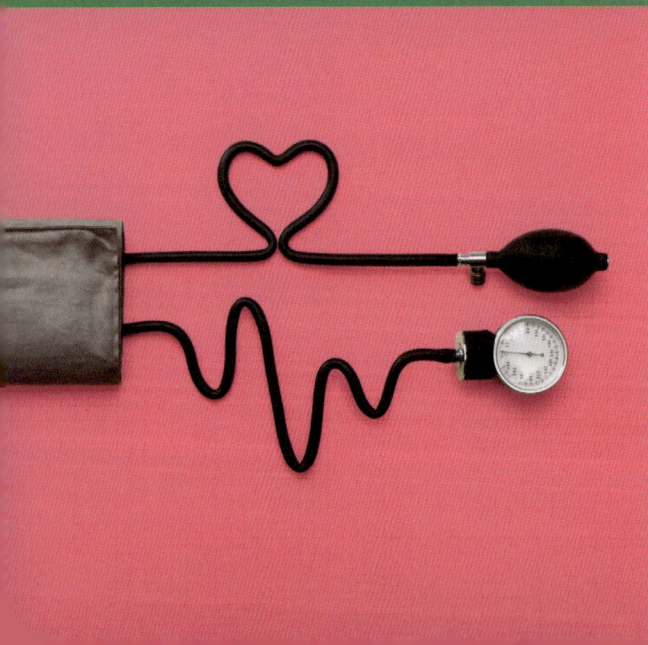

What to Do

Today, set the stage for a better night's sleep. First, consider installing blackout shades, as research shows that adults exposed to light when they sleep may be more likely to develop high blood pressure than those who sleep in complete darkness. Next, find a spot to charge your phone that's not in your bedroom so blue light and scrolling won't keep you up. Finally, try to crash between 10 p.m. and 11 p.m.—a study found that people who fell asleep within this window had a lower rate of developing cardiovascular disease than those who conked out earlier or later.

30 Monday

1 Tuesday ◑

2 Wednesday

3 Thursday

4 Friday Hanukkah Begins

5 Saturday

6 Sunday

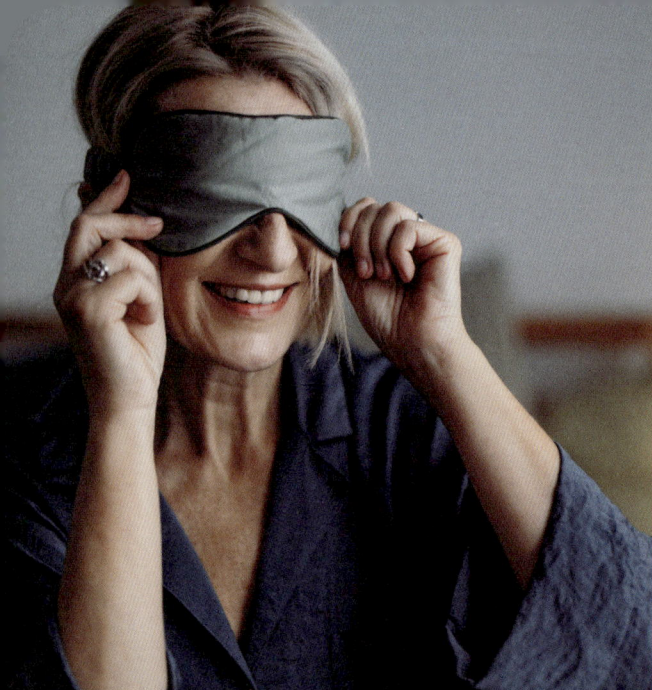

December 7–13

2026

M	T	W	T	F	S	S
	1	2	3	4	5	6
7	8	9	10	11	12	13
14	15	16	17	18	19	20
21	22	23	24	25	26	27
28	29	30	31			

ADDRESS SLEEP APNEA

Getting deep, restorative sleep supports brain health in a variety of ways, from consolidating memories to actively removing toxins from the brain. But one sleep disruptor people often miss is sleep apnea, which affects roughly 39 million American adults, says Zaldy S. Tan, M.D., M.P.H., director of the Memory & Healthy Aging Program at Cedars-Sinai.

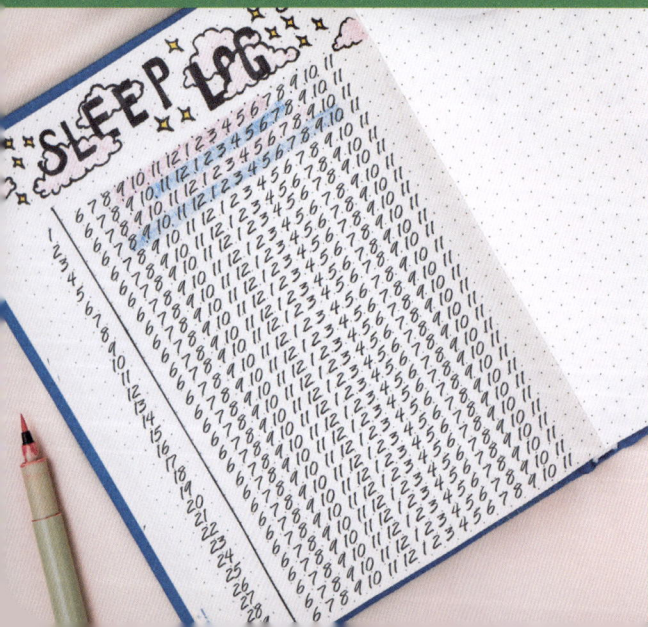

What to Do

Sleep apnea occurs when your airway gets temporarily obstructed while you're asleep, resulting in reduced airflow. This means not enough oxygen is getting to your brain, causing you to gasp for air. If you have a partner, they'll be able to spot signs like loud snoring and stop-start breathing, gasping, or choking in the middle of the night. If you sleep alone, take note of increased daytime sleepiness, frequent night awakenings, and morning headaches, and consider wearing a sleep tracker. Talk to your doctor if you show signs of sleep apnea. The sooner the condition is diagnosed, the better off you'll be.

7 Monday

8 Tuesday

9 Wednesday ●

10 Thursday

11 Friday

12 Saturday

13 Sunday

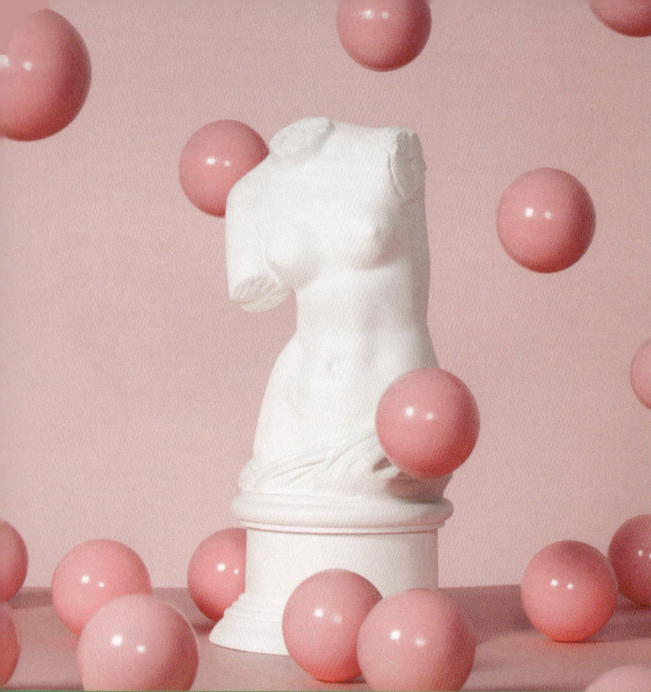

December
14–20

2026

M	T	W	T	F	S	S
	1	2	3	4	5	6
7	8	9	10	11	12	13
14	15	16	17	18	19	20
21	22	23	24	25	26	27
28	29	30	31			

KNOW MORE ABOUT MENOPAUSE

Menopause used to be treated like an illness, but it's not one. That said, when you're postmenopausal you no longer benefit from the protective effects of estrogen, raising your risk of health issues you may not have had to think about before, including mood changes. If you feel your life has changed significantly, talk with your doctor about treatment options.

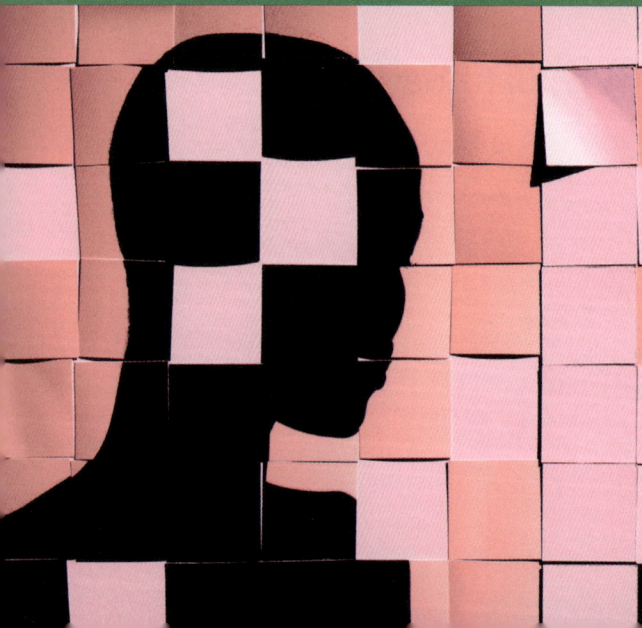

What We Know

Studies suggest that up to 68% of perimenopausal women report heightened depressive symptoms (compared with around a third of premenopausal women). Some women may become mildly irritable, while others suddenly feel sad or anxious or experience full-blown depression even if they've never had mental health struggles before. If you're feeling depressed or anxious, let your doctor know. The Menopause Society guidelines recommend psychotherapy and/or antidepressants and note that for some women, hormone therapy may help.

14 Monday

15 Tuesday

16 Wednesday

17 Thursday ◐

18 Friday

19 Saturday

20 Sunday

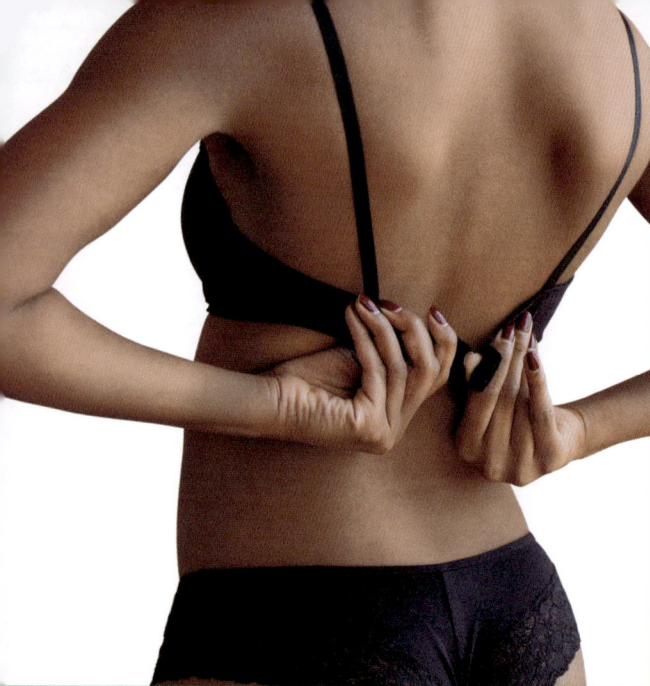

December 21–27

2026

M	T	W	T	F	S	S
		1	2	3	4	5	6
7	8	9	10	11	12	13
14	15	16	17	18	19	20
21	**22**	**23**	**24**	**25**	**26**	**27**
28	29	30	31			

DON'T WORRY ABOUT BREAST SELF-EXAMS

Those plastic shower tag reminder cards are a thing of the past. "We learned through large research studies that teaching women to do self breast exam didn't reduce breast cancer mortality. Most women didn't do it even when told to." says Susan Brown, R.N., senior director of health information and publications at Susan G. Komen.

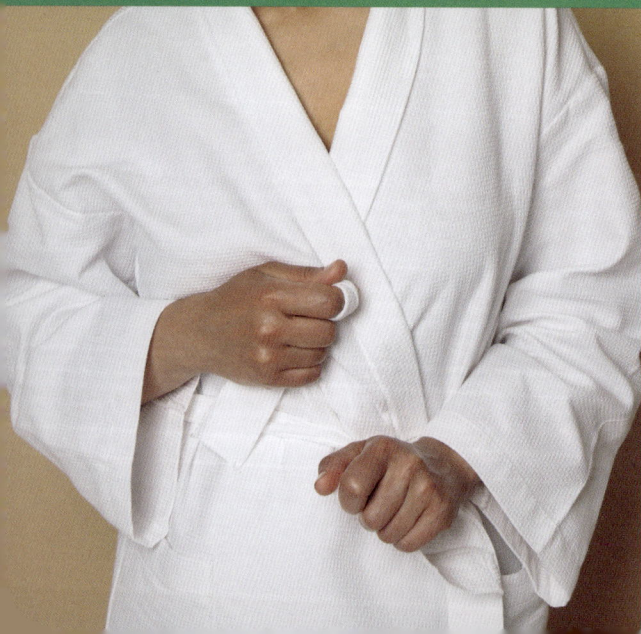

What We Know

The old-school breast self-exam you may have been told to do may no longer be an official ask, but that doesn't mean you should ignore your breasts. "What we have found is that women notice breast changes in the shower or when dressing, or a partner notices. Being familiar with your breasts is what's important," says Brown.

Take some time to get to know how they look and feel, and keep in mind that it's normal for there to be slight changes during your monthly cycle as well as throughout your life. However, if you notice anything that seems out of the ordinary, don't just stay home and worry about it, says Brown. See a doctor.

21 Monday First Day of Winter

22 Tuesday

23 Wednesday

24 Thursday ○ Christmas Eve

25 Friday Christmas Day

26 Saturday Kwanzaa Begins

27 Sunday

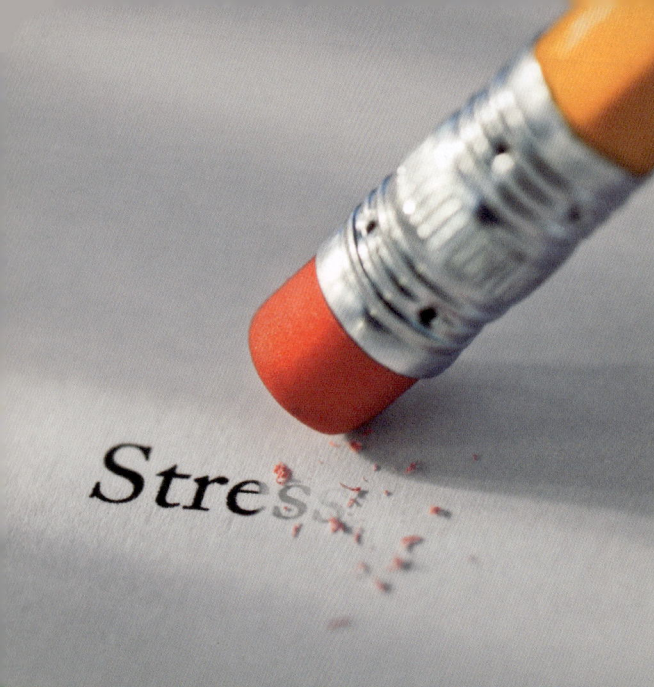

December 28–January 3

2026-2027

M	T	W	T	F	S	S
	1	2	3	4	5	6
7	8	9	10	11	12	13
14	15	16	17	18	19	20
21	22	23	24	25	26	27
28	29	30	31	1	2	3

TAKE TIME TO DE-STRESS

Remembering to take a few minutes to pause when you're feeling stressed is one of the fastest ways to find your road to calm. There are dozens of solutions to just about any problem you face, so giving your brain and body a moment to relax and process what you're experiencing can give the space you need to see things anew and form a quick plan.

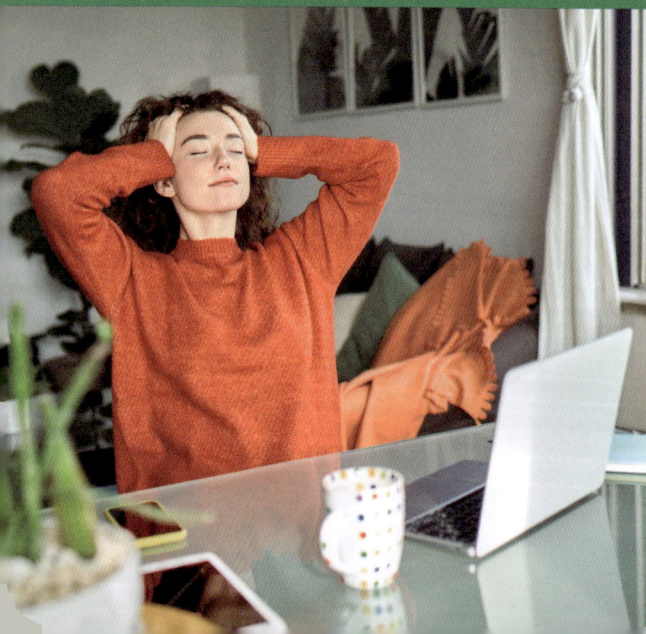

Why It Works

When you're stressed and anxious, cortisol (a stress hormone) runs high, which has an impact on the hippocampus as well as other sections of the brain that are involved in memory, research has found. So, for example, if you can't remember where you stashed your phone and are frantically flipping over the couch cushions, instead take a break, sit down on that couch, and breathe deeply for a minute or two. When your brain calms down, you'll be much better able to focus on your next steps—and reclaim the sense of peace you so richly deserve.

28 Monday

29 Tuesday

30 Wednesday ◑

31 Thursday New Year's Eve

1 Friday New Year's Day

2 Saturday

3 Sunday

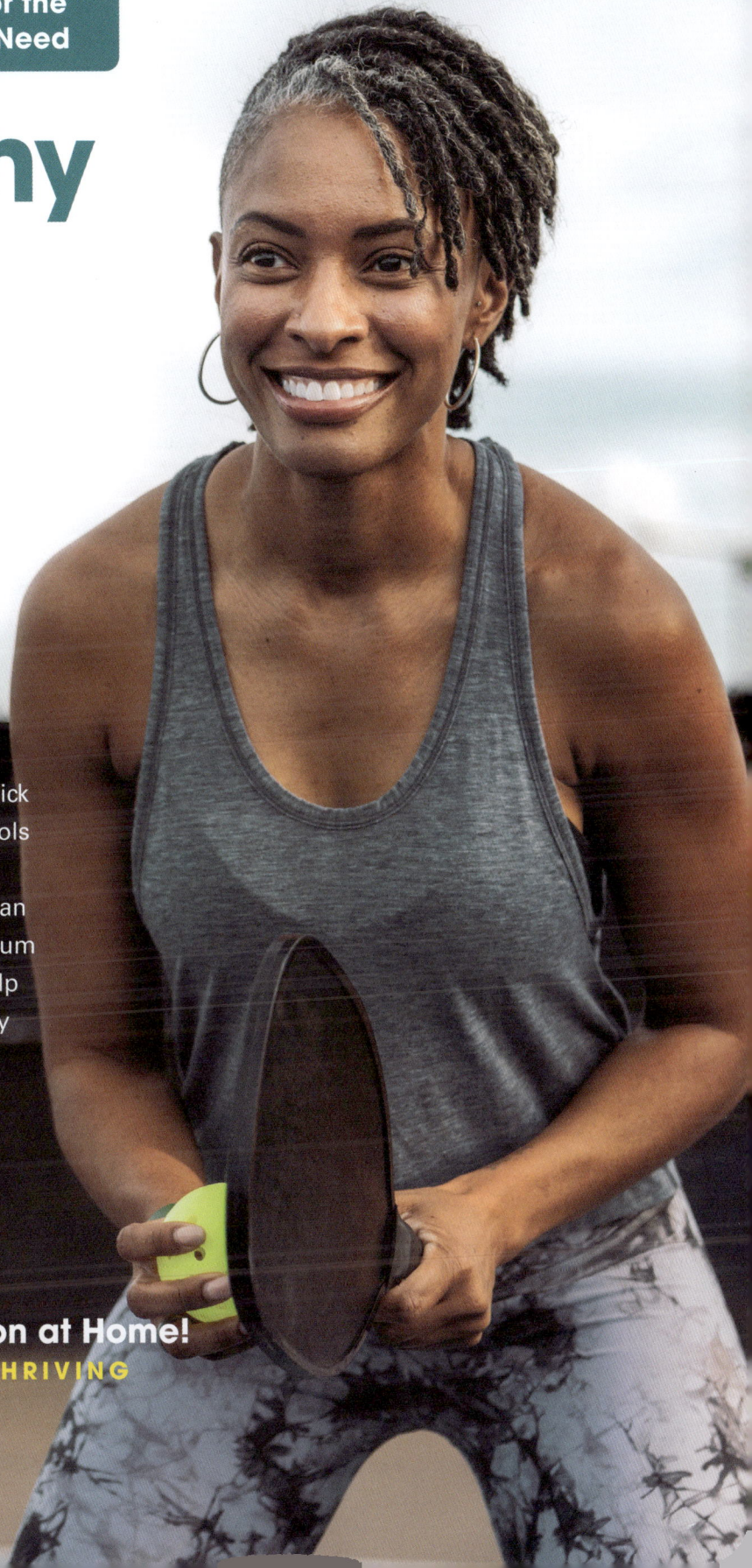

PHOTO CREDITS

(All Left to Right/Top to Bottom)